ROUNDWORK GUIDES

Series Editor
Jane Springer

GROUNDWORK GUIDE

Sex for Guys

Manne Forssberg

Groundwood Books
House of Anansi Press

Toronto Berkeley

Translated by
Maria Lundin

Groundwood Books / House of Anansi Press
110 Spadina Avenue, Suite 801, Toronto, Ontario M5V 2K4
Distributed in the USA by Publishers Group West
1700 Fourth Street, Berkeley, CA 94710

We acknowledge for their financial support of our publishing
program the Canada Council for the Arts, the Government of
Canada through the Book Publishing Industry Development
Program (BPIDP) and the Ontario Arts Council.

 ONTARIO ARTS COUNCIL
CONSEIL DES ARTS DE L'ONTARIO

Library and Archives Canada Cataloguing in Publication
Forssberg, Manne
Sex for guys / Manne Forssberg ; translated by Maria Lundin.
Translation of: Kukbruk — en bok om kärlek, känslor och kön för
unga killar och andra undrande.
(Groundwork Guides)
Includes bibliographical references and index.
ISBN-13: 978-0-88899-770-8 (bound)
ISBN-13: 978-0-88899-771-5 (pbk.)
ISBN-10: 0-88899-770-1 (bound)
ISBN-10: 0-88899-771-X (pbk.)
1. Sex instruction for men. 2. Men — Sexual behavior. 3. Sex
(Psychology).
I. Lundin, Maria II. Title.
HQ36.F6613 2007   306.7081   C2007-904285-6

Design by Michael Solomon
Printed and bound in Canada

Contents

This book is dedicated to Minna, my youngest sister. Carefully, we'll turn the world in the right direction.

Foreplay

I bet there are things that you'd really like to know about sex but you feel like you don't have anyone to ask. Why is one of your testicles bigger than the other? How do you know if a girl has an orgasm? And how fast should you thrust when you're having intercourse? How do you break up? Can you have sex when your girlfriend has her period? How is a guy supposed to act in bed? These are the types of questions I try to answer in this book.

This guidebook is partly about factual things to do with sex and love. Like what part is where on a vagina, what year porn became legal, and what those weird spots on your dick are. But this book is also about relationships, infatuations and having sex. I talk about my own experiences, and other young guys and girls answer questions about their experiences. (I say "girls," but I'm really talking about young women. It's one of those sexist things that guys are guys, and sound like adults, no matter what their age, but women are often girls. It's a bad habit, but it's hard to change.) Sometimes I give advice, but often there's no one piece of advice that's right for everyone. Think of this book as your partner in a conversation. No thoughts or feelings are prohibited here — all thoughts and feelings are okay.

One more thing. Some people think they know exactly who you are because you're young and you're a guy. Some might think you're technically inclined. Others might think that you can't keep your hands off girls. I know one thing: I don't know you. You could be anyone. That's why this book is about a whole range of different sexual facts, feelings and behaviors, so as many readers as possible can have their questions answered. You can choose to read this book from beginning to end, or you can jump around randomly and focus on specific things you want to learn about. The idea behind this book is to talk about things you might not be willing to bring up with your parents, your teachers, or even your friends.

Chapter 1
Penis

In a typical urban landscape, phallic shapes line up as far as the eye can see — light posts, church steeples, high-rises, chimneys, antennae. All these phalluses reach and stretch up into the sky as humans walk around below toting their cigars, ice creams and huge camera lenses. Our world is filled with phallic symbols, in various shapes, sizes and varieties.

Personally, I love having a penis. Yes, it can be a pain. Sometimes it gets squished into an uncomfortable position in your pants, and it always stands up at the worst times. It can be a shrunken raisin, a steel rod, something in between and much, much more.

A penis has many shapes. Mine has taken hundreds of different forms, often several in one day. The penis's changeability is part of its magic. I can pee with my penis but also use it for pleasure; it can bring me and others joy. Sometimes it puts on the amazing spectacle of ejaculation, pulling itself into a kind of muscle spasm, totally out of my control, then suddenly spilling over — just as impressive every time.

Penis semantics are often confusing. Should we call it cock, dick, weenie, willie, wiener, peter or manhood? In this book, we'll mostly use penis to keep it simple and straightforward, but dick is catchy, too, so I may throw that one in if I need to change it up.

The Importance of Size

Of course size matters. A huge 40-inch TV screen is nicer to watch than a little 13-inch set, a big apartment is roomier than a small one, and tiny lapdogs are way more annoying than big dogs. But with penises, it's different. There's really no point in having a massive tool. And even small models can work miracles.

Through the ages and all over the planet, men have worried about their penis size. The eternal question is, "Do I have a normal-sized penis?" In other words, "Am I good enough?" I've heard and read tons of similar questions from worried guys. In some cases, they're terrified their partner is going to leave them because they're too small, even though their penises are average in length. In fact, most of us probably worry about what we've got between our legs.

There's no doubt that we live in a competitive world where everything is measured, compared and evaluated. Measuring penises in the locker room is commonplace, and lots of guys worry that small penises will mean dissatisfaction in the bedroom. Many guys stubbornly refuse to accept that size isn't all-important, so they're destined to walk around obsessed and anxiety-ridden about it.

In English, when you're talking about a brave, strong man, you say, "He's got balls." In Swedish, you say, "He has a boner," when a guy distinguishes himself. In Bolivia, the Laymi people say, "He has a fantastic penis," to describe someone who has achieved something really major. A Ferrari comes with more status than a Lada — and so does a big dick. Don't forget, though, that a penis can be very different in size when it's flaccid and when it's erect. Some people are "growers" (small when flaccid but large when erect) and some are "showers" (large when flaccid but small when erect).

It's easy to get a distorted image of your own penis. You're always seeing it from above, a perspective that makes it look small.

You look at other penises in the change room and you think they all look pretty big. But chances are the guy you're looking at feels small when he looks at you, while you're torturing yourself about his superiority in the penis department. Everyone's penis looks different from up top: it's as if your penis disappears into itself.

There are girls who prefer big dicks, just like there are girls who prefer small ones. But I don't think any girl is so into the big variety that she can't appreciate a moderately sized penis. On the other hand, guys who are extremely well hung can have serious problems with women. For obvious reasons, sex can be really painful. Anal sex is more difficult if you are really large, and it is much easier to suck a smaller specimen than it is to blow a big one.

So, yes, it's true. Size is really important — to all those men and boys who are worried about it. The longing for a bigger penis probably isn't as much about being a better lover as it is about impressing your sex partners and the other guys in the locker room. Having a big dick has always been seen as "manly." But most of us know, deep down, that you don't become a better lover by having a bigger dick. Besides, you don't get more sex because you're well-endowed. Your size only becomes obvious once you take your pants off, and by then you're already in a pretty intimate situation. No one ever changes their mind because of someone's penis size.

Anyhow, sex is about so much more than penetration. Sex is caressing, kissing, touching, licking and — well, the list goes on and on. It can be a big turn-off if a guy lacks confidence and hates his own penis. Being with someone who is content with himself is always the sexiest thing of all.

So love your penis and marvel over its transformational powers. Hold your dick and be happy about how good it feels. Have a pee and be in awe of how fantastically nature has arranged everything down there. In the penis department, we live in the best of all worlds. No doubt about it.

Leonardo, 17

I think guys care more than girls about big cocks. Everyone is always comparing in the shower. They're all pretty small when they're limp, and yet, the guy who has the biggest flaccid cock wins. He's the man, the king of the shower. I'm sort of medium, but a buddy of mine from high school had a massive one, it was crazy big and really thick — the thing looked like a baseball bat.

Tanya, 21

I don't think dick size is very important. The size doesn't determine how good it feels. You can be just as satisfied with a big one or a small one.

When I was younger I was so intensely fascinated with penises in general that I didn't even think about size. But I have been in situations where size actually did matter.

One time I met a guy on a trip to Thailand and I slept with him. He had such a huge penis that I couldn't breathe and I fainted when he entered me. So of course we had to stop. He pulled out really fast and tried to shake me awake. I came to and I had no idea what had happened. It was so incredibly weird.

With a really big cock, you have to have much longer foreplay to make it work well and feel nice. I think it's important to take it easy and check in with your partner if you have a big penis.

Some guys I know who have really small penises still manage to satisfy their girlfriends vaginally. You can give your partner pleasure whether you're big or small.

Besides, the penis isn't the only instrument of pleasure. A lot of guys seem to think that the penis and the size are so incredibly important. But not everything is about the dick and how you use it. There are lots of other things to do.

Peter, 17

Sometimes, dick size is really important. It varies on a daily basis. Almost all guys probably wish they had a bigger penis sometimes. Some really well-endowed guys I know think having a big dick is a real drag because they can never have normal sex. If you had to choose between a really big one and a really small one, you'd probably regret it either way. Having a ten-incher would be kind of fun, I guess. I think guys are the most hung up about penis size; girls probably prefer smaller penises.

Your Guided Dicktour

Hi and welcome to a breathtaking journey inside a man's underwear! Fasten your seatbelts and prepare yourself for today's dicktour. Let's head down to the most exciting part of the male groin: the penis. If you have questions, just put up your hand and I'll answer them one at a time.

First comes the most difficult leg of our entire journey: the pubic hair. Follow me, single file, and make sure not to get lost as we pass through this dense and impenetrable jungle. Finally, we reach the root of the penis. This is where our dickadventure starts. Let's stop here for a breather after that grueling pubic-hair hike before we move on.

From here we can see down the penis shaft, with the glans — also called the head of the penis — down at the far end. Follow me and we'll go have a look. You'll notice as we find our way down the shaft that the skin on the penis has no fat underneath it. That's why you can see the sebaceous glands and veins so clearly. (The sebaceous glands produce fat, or sebum, that lubricates the surface of the penis.)

Now we're arriving at the glans. If you're circumcised, your glans is fully exposed. At the very tip of the glans you'll see the urethral meatus, the hole where urine comes out. A ridge of skin called the corona (the crown) separates the glans and the shaft of the penis. Take a look underneath the glans and you'll see a thin strip of skin at the edge of the corona called the frenum or frenulum. When you have an erection, the frenum contracts a little so the glans is pulled down. On circumcised guys, the frenum is often — but not always — the most sensitive part of the penis.

If you're uncircumcised, there's just a small part of the glans peeking out from under the foreskin. On uncircumcised guys, the entire glans or head is very sensitive — it is actually the male equivalent to the clitoris. Underneath the foreskin, there is a gland that produces protective fat which is specially designed to prevent friction between the glans and the inside of the foreskin. Help me pull the foreskin back so we can have a closer look. That sticky white stuff you see (and maybe smell) is that fatty secretion I mentioned earlier. The official name is smegma, but it's often just called headcheese. Anyone know why? That's right — because it smells and feels kind of like cheese. There's still some scientific debate about whether headcheese is beneficial or not. But there's one thing everyone agrees on — when smegma is allowed to accumulate, it is of no use whatsoever. Rinsing the area with warm water is the best way to guard against accumulation. Some scientists say that you should avoid using soap on the glans because it depletes your natural oils, but it's perfectly fine to wash it with water. This penis hasn't seen water for a little while... hence the smell.

If you look closely at the base of the glans, you'll see some white spots on the corona. No, they're not dangerous, they're actually really common — but lots of guys worry about them. The official name for these white spots is pearly penile papules, but they're nothing more than harmless skin irregularities. About 70 percent of all men have these spots; they usually show up during adolescence, but change in size, number and color over time.

Now let's head over and check out the scrotum. Why does it hang loose like that outside the body? Well, because the scrotum works like a natural air-conditioning system. Since the rest of the body is at 37°C (99°F), and a temperature of 34°C (93°F) is needed to properly produce and maintain sperm, the scrotum keeps a healthy distance from the body to stay cooler.

If you look closely you will notice that the scrotum is constantly moving up and down. No, it's not trying to communicate with us. It moves because of these heat-sensitive muscles called tunica dartos. When it's hot, the scrotum stretches out to increase the surface area of the skin for greater heat evaporation; when it's cold, it shrinks to get closer to the body and minimize the evaporation surface. The blood is also cooled on its way into the scrotum to help maintain the right temperature. Pretty smart, some say. I say it's brilliant.

Inside the scrotum you'll find two testicles, each with an epididymus and a vas deferens or deferent duct. The testicles' job is to produce sperm. You're probably wondering if it's abnormal to have two different-sized balls. No — on the contrary, most men have two different-sized testicles. Looking closer, you'll notice that they also hang at different heights. That's probably so they don't bump into each other all the time.

A healthy man produces about 1,800 sperm per second. Once the sperm is formed, it empties into the epididymus, which functions kind of like a wine cellar. Once there, the sperm is stored while it matures. It takes about seventy-two to seventy-five days from the time the sperm is formed until it's ready to be used. The epididymus is connected to the vas deferens, which transports the fully matured sperm to the urethra, where it mixes with other fluids to become semen before it is shot out of the body as an ejaculation.

Well, my friends, that's all I have to say on this subject. Any questions? What was that? Morning boners? Ah, yes, good question, very good question. Lots of guys are confused about why their penis insists on getting stiff when they wake up and need to pee. And it makes it hard to pee, too, doesn't it? Partly because it's hard to steer and partly because it's hard to pee when you have an erection.

When we dream, the body relaxes in the same way as it does when we're sexually aroused, and your penis responds in the same way too — you get an erection. If you dream right before waking up, the erection often remains. If your bladder is full, the effect is even stronger, because your bladder pushes against the nerves that control the erectile muscles.

Bent Dicks

A penis can, as I mentioned, vary in size. But it can also vary in shape, color and appearance. Men the world over write in to sex columnists asking about their off-center or bent penises. Is something wrong with me? Will I be able to have sex with this left hook? Am I handicapped?

Just stay calm. Actually, a completely straight penis is really unusual. You'll either bend to the left or the right, although the left bend is most common. Back when people still had their clothes sewn by a tailor, the tailor even took into account which direction the penis pointed in!

Even if you have a banana or a lop-sided sausage, intercourse works just fine. The only time there might be a problem is when the bend is over thirty degrees, when you have painful erections or when intercourse is impossible because of the curvature. But most likely, even these issues can be fixed with easy adjustments during sex. Penises aren't made of stone and neither are vaginas. Which is why, as weird as it might seem, bent penises are as good as the straighter ones.

Male Circumcision

If you are a circumcised man, it means you have had your foreskin removed. Usually the foreskin is cut or snipped off in babyhood, but sometimes the surgery is performed during adulthood, most often for religious or cultural reasons.

In many religions and cultures, Judaism and Islam for example, male circumcision is standard. In North America, doctors started doing non-religious circumcision during the late 1800s, and today, about 60 percent of North American men are still routinely circumcised. One of the now-outdated reasons for circumcising boys in the last century was to make masturbation more difficult, since self-pleasure of any kind was often considered to be sinful.

The skin on the glans of a circumcised man thickens and hardens, and some of the nerve cells found in the foreskin disappear. Some claim that circumcised men have fewer problems with premature ejaculation since they have a less sensitive glans. Others are against circumcision precisely because they claim that the circumcised man's sex life is negatively affected by the loss of the foreskin.

Circumcision can also be a good remedy if your foreskin is too tight. Before puberty, it's not a problem if you can't pull your foreskin up over the glans. It has its own cleaning system and doesn't need to be washed. But when adolescence arrives, that function disappears and guys have to clean the glans on their own. There's also an increase in the production of sweat and oil secretions during puberty — and more smegma — so it becomes important to be able to pull the foreskin back. And it's not just a question of hygiene. It's impossible to have a functioning sex life if your foreskin is too tight. You can't masturbate or perform penetration. And sometimes, if the ring of the foreskin is too tight and not able to retract during an erection, it can cause fluid buildup and swelling.

Dick Control

If you're worried about how your penis is doing, schedule an exam with your family doctor or at a clinic. Checking the status of your penis is usually quick and painless. The medical visit is also a great opportunity to pick up condoms, make sure that all is well with your genitals, and have a chat with someone who knows a lot about these things.

Personally, I was really impressed by my first genital exam. Of course, I was very nervous and wondered how it would go. I worried about all kinds of things. What if I got a boner? What if I farted? I didn't fart or get a boner, but even if I had, it would have been totally fine. Nurses and doctors can handle pretty much anything. I chose to be examined by a female doctor. She touched my penis so calmly and professionally that it felt like she was grabbing my shoulder or something.

A genital exam often starts with a chat. The doctor, nurse or specialist asks questions to figure out who you are sexually and what issues you are dealing with. Then you're asked to pull your pants down and lie down on an examination table. While you're lying there, try to just relax and stay calm. The person examining you will point a bright light at your groin and then they'll get started. He/she will feel for the lymph glands in the pubic region. He/she will examine the scrotum, and look at the foreskin (if you're uncircumcised) and the skin on the shaft. Then, he/she will examine the urethral opening by separating it with his/her fingers. That's the basic exam, and it only takes a few minutes.

When you get tested for sexually transmitted infections (STIs), there are different methods for different types of diseases. You might need a blood test, a urine test, a urethral swab test (which entails squeezing some secretion from the urethra opening) or a test where they take a swab of suspect sores or blisters. See Chapter 10 for more details on STIs.

Dick on Strike

Almost all men are afflicted by impotence at some time or another. The penis refuses to stand up and stretch out. Usually it happens exactly when you least want it. The lack of an erection can have any number of explanations. Erectile problems can be the result of side effects from certain medications. Drinking can also make getting an erection more difficult. But for younger guys the most common reasons for impotence are probably pressure and stress. If you're nervous about performing during sex, it's common for your penis not to cooperate. And the next time, you might be even more nervous or stressed out, and the anxiety puts your penis out of commission yet again. Sometimes you might not even be aware that you're putting pressure on yourself, and it will seem unexplainable when your penis goes on strike. But erection problems are usually easy to cure. Sometimes a conversation with your partner is all it takes, or the problem will go away on its own. If you have repeated and continuous problems getting or keeping an erection, take advantage of all the sex support resources that are available online or by phone. You should consider getting a medical exam as well.

Chapter 2
Vagina

Phallic symbols definitely outnumber vaginal symbols in our society. But one big vaginal symbol that makes all the phallic stuff pale in comparison is the ocean. Infinite and deep, it makes all those radio towers and high-rises look painfully obvious, and the difference in size is laughable. Compared to almost anything else in the world, the ocean is wide, nourishing and full of life.

When I want to talk about female genitalia, I run out of good words really fast. Men seem to have an easier time naming their sexual organs than women do. (Unfortunately, this is probably just one more symptom of the inequality between men and women — there's more on this in Chapter 5.) Lots of girls still don't have a good word for one of their most important body parts — so they end up defaulting to "down there." Imagine if it was considered shameful to talk about your head and you blushed and felt compelled to say "up there" every time you talked about it.

I think that old "down there" thing is just terrible — it's not even a real word! Worse, it's an anti-word. It's high time we all started to feel okay about using the real V words. Twat, muff, beaver, mouse, vulva, pie, cunt, treasure, vag? What the heck should we call women's genitals? Vulva is alright, but it only describes the outer genitals and sounds kind of hippie erotic to me. Cunt sounds just a little too crass. And I think we can forget about beaver and mouse – it is a human body part after all. Vagina is probably the best word to describe the whole area, even though scientifically, it refers to one specific part of the inner female genitalia. We'll use vagina in this book in order to keep it simple and straightforward, but vag works, too, when we need some variety.

No two vaginas are alike. One gynecologist told me that she thinks that each vagina is as unique as a human face. But despite huge differences in appearance, every vagina shares, of course, the same general form and function.

Outer Genitals – The Vulva

We can divide the vagina into the inner and outer genitals. The outer genitals are those that are visible outside of a woman's body, and they are known as the vulva. Let's have a look.

Above the vaginal opening is the mons, a raised area of tissue over the pubic bone. If the girl in question has reached puberty, the mons is covered in pubic hair. It consists of fat cells and nerve endings that make it pleasurable to the touch. The fatty tissue also cushions the pubic bone during sexual intercourse.

Below the mons are the outer labia, which are also covered in hair. They are located alongside the inner labia, which often peek out from under the outer ones (depending on the size of each set). There are glands in between the inner and outer labia that produce vaginal discharge, or mucus, which is similar to the smegma that guys produce.

The inner labia surround and protect the vaginal and urethral openings. These fine folds of mucous membranes are totally hairless and contain lots of nerve endings, so they are very sensitive to the touch. The inner labia are usually closed and touch one another, but with arousal, they fill with blood, swell and separate. The size, length and color of the inner labia vary widely from woman to woman. They can be long and thick, or barely visible, and may look purple, red, pink, blackish or brown – all completely normal. Where the inner labia meet at the top, under the mons, they form the hood of the clitoris, which protects the clitoris. Its function is similar to that of the foreskin.

Many of us think that the clitoris (also known as the love button) is hidden and hard to find, but this supposed problem of locating the clit is a bit exaggerated. If you separate the inner labia a little and feel upwards with your finger until you get to where the inner labia meet at the top, you can feel something sticking out. That's the clitoris, which fills with blood when a girl is turned on. In fact, the clitoris gets an erection. The reason many of us are so concerned with finding the love button is that for many women, it's a great place to be touched. Some women think it's easy to get too much of a good thing, though, because the clitoris can be very sensitive, and they prefer to be caressed around the clit or have it stimulated by rubbing the clitoral hood.

Inner Genitals – The Vagina

The inner genitals are the genital organs that are inside a woman's body. The vaginal canal is one of these, and consists of a series of folds. In an adult woman, the average length of the vaginal canal is 8 to 10 centimetres (3 to 4 inches), but it is highly flexible and stretches like an accordion during sexual arousal. The vaginal opening sits slightly above where the inner labia meet at the perineum (the area between the vulva and the anus).

About half an inch inside the vaginal opening is the hymen, which is made up of several folds of mucous membrane. In young girls, the hymen is quite tight, closing off the vaginal opening, but the older a woman is, the more flexible and elastic the hymen becomes. The thickness of the hymen also varies from person to person. The hymen is what causes some girls to bleed during their first sexual intercourse. But it's not true that all girls bleed the first time. Fewer than half of all women bleed the first time they have sex, and the majority of women do not experience pain.

To have intercourse, the vaginal opening must be wet. The

moisture that is normally present at the vaginal opening is not enough. When a woman is aroused, the vaginal walls start producing a lubricating secretion. It can happen at any time, kind of like an erection. A bumpy bus ride or an exciting thought can be enough to make the vagina wetter. How wet you get depends on the degree of arousal, but it can also vary from person to person. This lubrication makes it easier to penetrate the vagina. Without lubrication, penetration can be painful, especially for the girl but also for the guy. In the worst case scenario, you can injure the vagina.

Right at the top of the vaginal canal is the cervix, which sort of dips down into the vagina. (If you touch the cervix gently with your finger, it feels a lot like the tip of your nose.) During penetration, you can sometimes bump into the cervix with your penis, which can be painful for the girl, so you need to be careful. In the middle of the cervix is the os, the narrow entrance to the uterus, which connects the vagina and the uterus. It serves the important function of allowing menstrual blood and secretions out of the uterus, and, as part of the reproductive process, transporting sperm in and babies out.

Lastly, between the clitoris and the vaginal opening you'll find the opening to the urethra, where urine exits the body.

Menstruation

It happens to all girls. One day, they get their period. Most commonly, it makes its entrance around age twelve to fourteen (but it can arrive earlier or later, too). Some girls long for this sign of womanhood; others think it's a pain or find it embarrassing. In terms of sexual development, a girl getting her period can be compared to a guy starting to ejaculate. Suddenly you're capable of making a baby. In some ways, you're now a grownup. For some girls, the experience of getting their period can be mysterious and strange. In the past, before sex ed, girls were often terrified when their first period started. Imagine how you would react if you suddenly started bleeding from your penis. Terror would probably just be the first in a series of bad feelings!

There are two common variations to the reactions girls have when they get their first period. Some girls feel grown-up, relieved and proud. This type of girl takes pleasure in buying pads and discussing tampons with her friends. Other girls think getting their period is a drag or just really embarrassing. Maybe she's the first to get it in her class, and she's the only one having to deal with what's happening to her body. Maybe she's miserable because her period is the first sign she'll have to give up on her dream of becoming a professional baseball player. Or maybe she has brutal period cramps and has to take days off from school. Most girls don't talk to guys very much about their period. Comments like "This weekend I had my first period. Isn't that fantastic, baby? I'm a woman now!" are unfortunately just not that common.

Since first-hand information is hard to come by, it's easy for myths to spread among guys. Some think that girls go crazy or become aggressive when they have their period. Others walk around trying to figure out which girls have their period at a given time. "Maybe Lisa, she seems a little irritable," they reason, thinking they know it all. More likely than not, Lisa is mad because she screwed up the latest math test, or because she missed the rim shot in yesterday's gym class.

Some girls do have severe pre-menstrual symptoms – which may include physical and emotional symptoms such as headache, fatigue, cravings, depression and crying spells. Girls and women who suffer from pre-menstrual syndrome or PMS are in the minority, however. In fact, it's really hard to tell if a girl has her period or not. If you absolutely need to keep track of a girl's period for some reason, the most reliable sign is that she might complain about pain and be excused to go to the school nurse for medication. The other changes that can come with menstruation just aren't visible. Some bodily changes might happen a few days before a girl gets her period, when her body is getting ready. The hormones that cause menstruation might cause a girl's breasts to swell or her body to retain more water. The extra hormones can cause some women to become more emotional or irritable during this time. Others are less affected and don't experience mood changes.

It is crucial never to make assumptions about girls and their periods or to catch yourself saying, for example, "You must be on the rag or something" or "Are you PMS-ing?" It might make her feel like you've punched her in the stomach or thrown a bucket of cold water over her. These kinds of statements can lead to embarrassment, anger or even revenge. Few questions can make a person feel so mad or misunderstood. And after all, guys and girls need to understand each other. If you notice that a girl is feeling a little down, you can simply ask her how she's feeling — and then listen respectfully to what she tells you.

Sex During Menstruation

Girls and guys can often talk more openly about the girl's period in intimate situations. But you need to consider a few questions first. Can you have intercourse during her period? Does she even want to have sex during her period? Is sex during a girl's period gross?

To start with: sex during menstruation is safer than at other times, but it is still possible for a girl to get pregnant when she's menstruating. It is probably more unusual to have sex during menstruation in a casual relationship than it is in a committed relationship. Some girls feel bloated or otherwise uninterested in making out or having sex when they have their period, so they'd rather just hang out and watch a movie. Others feel extra horny during their period and don't care about a little blood. You'll be wearing a condom anyway, of course, so for those of you who might be worried about blood on your penis, the condom is excellent protection. It's worth thinking ahead about the fact that it can be kind of messy. You can handle it in a few different ways:

1) Don't worry about it.

2) Put a towel down to protect the sheets.

3) Change the sheets when you're done.

Overall, having sex with someone who has their period is pretty much the same as having sex with someone who's not.

Menstruation: How It Works

Menstruation is simply one phase of a cycle that the female body goes through each and every month. Two weeks before the period begins, the ovum, or egg, that resides in one of the two ovaries has matured enough that it is ready to move down into the fallopian tubes. Next, it travels to the uterus. (Keep in mind, pregnancy can occur during the journey down the fallopian tube, too.)

In the uterus, a nourishing, blood-filled mucous membrane forms once a month, providing a place for the egg to mature and grow if it is fertilized. If the egg is not fertilized, the mucous membrane is rejected from the uterus. That's where menstrual blood comes from. The period starts about two weeks after the egg descends from the ovary during what's called ovulation.

The entire process is called the menstrual cycle. The menstrual cycle is counted from the first day of the period to the first day of the next period. On average, the cycle is twenty-eight days long, but it can also be longer or shorter. Girls who have just started menstruating can have pretty irregular cycles, which is perfectly normal. The period itself usually lasts between three days and a week.

Women who are seriously underweight often don't get their period. If a woman's body is in starvation mode, hormone production doesn't work properly and ovulation doesn't occur. When a girl goes back to a normal weight, ovulation will start again.

Chapter 3
Kisses

When I was around twelve or so, I remember thinking that truth or dare was the best game ever. At that age, the favorite dare was a kiss. That's how I got my first kiss. We hid in the closet of the basement rec room. It was a bit clammy and alien, but still, it was great. We tried to kiss like we'd seen in the movies, crammed in there between winter coats, suitcases and old photo albums.

Unfortunately, truth or dare seemed a bit lame once grade six was over, and suddenly, we had to figure out for ourselves how to get kissed. And how did you do that? By walking up to someone and just planting a big, fat kiss on them in broad daylight? Or did you prearrange it somehow? I had no idea. I wasn't too worried about actual kissing technique, but how was I supposed to know if someone wanted my tongue in her mouth or not?

When the worst period of anxiety and waiting was over, I realized the problem was almost starting to resolve itself. From time to time, I got to kiss someone and each time, I became a bit surer of myself. Later I couldn't even remember how it happened – it was like kissing took on a life of its own. An amazing new world had opened up before me and it was just heaven to lie around, touching someone with their tongue in my mouth.

The First Kiss

Anna, 17

My first kiss felt weird. Not at all like I had imagined it. Mostly it was wet, slobbery and unpleasant. It was a regular day when I was in grade six, and it was with my first boyfriend. We were playing truth or dare. So then we started kissing a lot because we thought that's what going out was all about.

We were together for maybe a week after that, and then it was on to the next boyfriend. Grade six was like that for me.

Tommy, 19

My first kiss probably wasn't the best technically speaking, but it was hot and romantic. It was on my best friend's eighteenth birthday. We were at a party, and we held each other and had an amazing night until it was time to go home. It felt great. I ended up being really in love with her and we started going out after that.

How do you find someone to kiss?

If you're at a party and you know who you want to kiss, the trick is to keep close. Not by hanging around incessantly as if you're the person's bodyguard. Leeches don't get kissed. But find some way to show that you're interested – and keep in mind that clever pick-up lines work better in the movies than in real life. At the beginning, eye contact is the most important thing. If the looks start getting more intense, you will feel it in your stomach. And when you feel that buzz in your stomach, a kiss is the next logical step.

If the person you're checking out just looks irritated or gives you the one-finger salute, it's a good idea to put your kissing plans on the back burner. But if you can detect some sort of interest in the way he or she is looking at you, move bravely onward!

Dancing is another really good way to get things started. On the dance floor, people tend to relax their inhibitions and you can get in closer without seeming unnatural. Most kisses start with a hug, which is why slow dances are so perfect.

If you don't feel like dancing, or if the object of your affection doesn't feel like it either, there are other methods. Start a conversation. Give a compliment. Get close. If the person moves away from you every time you move closer, that's a bad sign. If it feels weird to start kissing in front of your friends, you can always suggest a walk. If it's cold, you can always warm each other up. Hopefully a kiss will be almost inevitable...

How do you let someone know you're interested?

John, 19
I'm not the most outwardly attractive guy. So I use my brain instead of my looks and it works pretty well. The crucial thing to nail is how to start talking to someone. After that, you can always charm them.

Angelica, 18
I'm pretty open so I'll just go up to anyone I'm interested in and start talking. It becomes pretty obvious if the person is just into talking about life and the weather or if he wants to make out. Then I'll take the initiative and throw myself at him. On the other hand, if I'm seriously into someone, I might be a bit more reserved so they don't think I'm a leech.

Ellen, 18
You should be at a dance or a concert or something. That way it's in the cards. If the vibe is good and there's music, you don't need to do much. Just check someone out, dance and start making out!

Neil, 16

Try to work some sexy subjects into the conversation, so both of you get a bit heated up.

Emily, 15

If I'm feeling forward, I'll just go up and say something like "Hey, are you available?" If I didn't get into those kinds of moods, I don't think much would ever happen — I would just obsess about the guys I'm interested in, since I'm actually kind of a coward.

How You Do It

Fast, slow, deep or shallow? Let's take it from the beginning. Kissing is about mouths touching and tongues meeting. The basic starting point for a kiss is mouth against mouth. If you both seem ready, then open your mouths and let your tongues touch and sort of circle each other. After that, it's all experimentation. What to do next usually becomes pretty obvious. It's important to remember that a kiss is not a one-man show. You're not running a race here. Try not to go too fast or hard right away — leave some time for both of you to feel your way. Kisses are about exploration and collaboration, like so much else when it comes to sex.

One of the most amazing things about kissing is that you're creating something together. It's like playing music with someone. When you listen to the other person, you find yourself playing in a way you could never have thought up on your own. It doesn't work if you just find a technique you like and then use it all the time. When a kiss is great, new things are always happening. A kiss can start as a peck, then become a slower, deeper kiss and then a faster, shallower kiss. Experiment away!

Do you have to be in love?

Some people think that kissing and love go together like coffee and cream. I take my coffee black, so I might not be the best person to answer this question, but I don't really agree. A kiss can mean a lot of things, but it can also be meaningless. Kisses may taste better when you're in love, but they can be really good even when you're not. Kissing someone doesn't mean you're in love or want to be with them forever — it doesn't even have to mean that you want to go out with the person. But of course, this varies from kiss to kiss. Kissing someone when it's just the two of you in broad daylight usually means more than kissing someone in the corner of a packed club. In short, it depends on the context.

But if you know that someone is in love with you, it's really crappy to kiss that person if you don't feel the same way. Take into consideration that people are fragile when they're in love. And if you promise to get in touch after the kiss, and you don't, that's just mean. Simply put, don't promise things you can't stick to and definitely don't lie in order to get kissed.

How do you want to be picked up?

Anna, 17

I want the person to walk up to me and just talk to me normally. I don't want them to suck up to me with compliments or stuff like that. It's great if they, like, ask if I want to hang out and suggest something fun to do together.

Petra, 17

It depends what the situation is. If it's just about picking me up for a make-out session, it works best to be pretty forward and persistent, but he has to be confident and good-looking to pull it off. The worst, though, is the sleazy close-talker guy, who whispers stuff like "Hey, wanna get it on?" And I hate it when guys touch me without asking. It's better if someone comes up with a big smile and says, "Wow, you're really hot, would it be cool if I came home with you later?" I like that attitude where you don't quite know if he's joking. Then it's easy to respond with a joke and keep each other guessing.

Chapter 4
Love

Love: A strong positive emotion of regard and affection.

Romantic relationships are basically a big mystery. Person X falls in love with person Y. Of all the people X knows, it's Y he's fallen in love with. That Y should fall in love with him, too, seems almost impossible, considering how many potential candidates exist in the world. And yet love is often answered with love. It happens again and again. People start relationships and go all crazy with love for each other.

Lots of young people believe that this far-fetched twist of fate will never happen to them. I thought that, too. But I was completely wrong. When I fell in love, it was as if I was totally changed. I forgot to eat and I needed almost no sleep. Everything centered on the person I was in love with. She was the last thing I thought about before falling asleep, and the first thing on my mind when I opened my eyes in the morning. I was so focused on her that I almost forgot all about me.

The feeling is often amazing, but sometimes sadness sneaks in, too. You can feel longing and torment if you don't see the person — like you're going to get sucked into a black hole. It's intense pleasure and pain at the same time.

Very few of us die without ever being in love or having a relationship. Love afflicts most humans. Imagine how much happiness romantic relationships have generated. And think about how much sadness and anxiety they have provided, too. If you were to add up all these feelings, they would be bigger than anything else in the world. Bigger than the amazement at the world's best guitar solo, the most successful invention or the hugest lottery winnings. Bigger than the anxiety about exams or fitting in or being successful.

In Love with Love

Sometimes it's like you're in love with everyone. In first period your heart pounds for your classmate at the next desk. The fire in your heart is the biggest in the country and you don't know what to do with all the warmth, horniness and nervous energy. At lunch, someone else makes you weak-kneed with attraction, and then at the bus stop, you see someone who makes you want to explode and fall on your knees to confess your love for them.

At home you're confused. Am I in love with everyone or no one? Maybe it was just that person in my class, or was it the one at the bus stop that I went most crazy for? Was the feeling strongest in my belly, my groin or my heart? Maybe you're really just in love with love. You're more infatuated with your own feelings than the people you're focusing your feelings on.

Being in love with love is neither a handicap nor a disease. Mostly, it's incredibly great. But when you're having a day like that, it can be a good strategy to keep some of those feelings to yourself. Declaring your love to fifteen different people in one day can turn out to be a little awkward. Someone could easily feel betrayed when they come across you writing love letters to a whole new set of people the next day.

How do you know when you're in love for real? Usually you feel it. A good sign is if there's a guy or a girl you always daydream about being close to and who you think about continuously. Being in love is like feeling everything at once. When you're around the person, you feel dizzy, tense, hot, horny or even a little miserable – or all of these at the same time.

Unrequited Love

All love has a streak of bad luck in it, but some love feels worse than almost anything else. When the person you're crazy about is making out with some idiot in the schoolyard, you want to die. It looks like they're eating each other, and you can feel the tears stinging your eyes and your body turning to mush as you watch them.

If there was a cure for feelings like that, I would put up a stand at the closest mall and give it away for free all day. But there isn't. I can't even share a decent method for coping with the experience.

What is important to know is that it does get better. It can take time, and until it happens you'll probably feel like you'll never be happy, calm and collected again – let alone fall in love with someone else. Usually people who are unhappily in love go through a period when they feel as if they are on negative auto-pilot. As soon as you spot someone you would normally check out, all you can think about is how much uglier and more useless she/he is compared to the person you're in love with.

Wallowing in misery and self-pity is fine for a while, but make sure you don't get stuck. At a certain point, you just have to get ready to head out there again to face the world. Some people start to get a strange pleasure out of torturing themselves. They spend their time thinking of themselves as unlovable losers, and imagining obsessively what their heart's desire is doing with his or her partner. In the long run, it's just not healthy. Try to stop thinking about them and open your eyes to others.

Once you're over your unrequited love, you'll find you're all the better for having gone through it. Pulling yourself out of all the sadness and emotional turmoil becomes an important part of your experience. You mature and grow and get ready to meet other fantastic people who are out there, waiting for you to fall in love all over again.

Love from Afar

Love doesn't have to be mutual to be happy, though. It can be enough to smell your love object's perfume from a distance to feel like the happiest person in the world. But if you're really in love you might get to a point where you want more than that. You want to be seen and liked and maybe start a relationship.

For a relationship to start, the feelings have to be mutual, and when you've been admiring someone from afar, you'll need to explore this person further before figuring out if that's the case or not. Stumbling up to someone on trembling legs in the cafeteria line can be terrifying or wonderful or both. It all depends on who you are as a person. If you're shy and prefer to avoid eye contact when you talk about your feelings, find a way that works for you. Messaging and texting have opened things up for all kinds of shy lovebirds.

Phase one is about getting closer to the person to figure out if it's possible that the feelings are mutual. This information is often the deciding factor. If you can't talk directly to the person you're in love with, it can be good to get to know one of their close friends.

Things that can be good to know if you're in love with someone at a distance:
- Their e-mail, cell phone number or messaging address.
- What online communities and chat rooms they hang out in.
- Their interests and hobbies.
- Whether or not they're single.

The more information you get, the easier it will be to make contact. Broad access to the Internet has revolutionized love and sex for people around the world. Cyberspace is amazing, since it can be a lot easier to start talking to your dream girl or dream boy there than in the hallways. When you've messaged each other, it will feel more natural to talk at school, at the mall or wherever your friends usually hang out.

The next step is to try to end up in the same places as the person you like. Find out what she/he is doing on Friday night or after school. If there's a party, make sure to get invited, and if she/he's in a sports tournament, drag your friends there. The more times you "bump into" the person, the bigger the chances that she/he will start noticing you and want to be near you, too.

But chance meetings and messaging might not feel like enough to you. Chemistry and feelings of infatuation might still remain and have nowhere to go. That's when it's time to suggest a date. Not necessarily an official super-romantic capital D date. A coffee, a walk in the park or just playing video games – these kinds of mini-dates aren't heavy or serious, so they won't make you so nervous.

Before long you'll sense whether your feelings are reciprocated or not, and then you'll be able to figure out what the next step should be. Or you'll discover your crush is great as a friend and you'll forget about being in love. It can go many ways. With love, there's no planning things out in advance.

Or, feel free to totally ignore all my advice. Maybe it's more your style to start the whole thing off with a big romantic serenade or an amazing kiss or a big dinner at your mom's house. There are no rules. As long as you don't treat anyone badly, anything goes. And remember, even if you "fail," going after someone you like always pays off: the more rejections you get, the more you learn about love. And the great love of your life may be your crush's best friend.

How do you make contact with the person you're in love with?

Angelica, 18
If I probably won't see the person again unless I make contact I'll be pretty forward and ask for a phone number. I generally call when I say I will, but I wait a day or two to create a little suspense.

Victor, 16
I make friends first and then I flirt a bit. Then I write a letter where I explain my feelings for the person. I'm very romantic, which I have realized is not always a good thing. I've been turned down three times because I was too passionate. They thought I was overly romantic. I say nice things and buy girls roses and stuff like that.

Ellen, 18
If someone gives me their phone number, I usually call. I start with small talk and then I explore by asking more concrete questions. But I think I'm kind of a coward. I really have to force myself to go up to someone. So it's easier for me when it's over the phone and I don't have to look the person in the eyes.

Sam, 16
I guess I try to be friends with the person first so we can get closer. If I think I want a relationship I take it very slowly. You start talking to the person you like, hang out for a while. But then you have to show that you want to be more than friends, otherwise everything can end up wrong and confused.

Making Yourself Over
You're crazy in love. Everything is about this one person, but she/he seems to have no idea you even exist. It's like they look right through you. At home you look at yourself in the mirror.

You look horrible. New pimples are showing up every day like red traffic lights and your clothes are ready for the second-hand store. And what's all that flab? My god, your breath smells like something died. Time for a change, you think. Hit the gym to tone up and head to the mall for new, cooler clothes. Maybe it's time for a personality tune-up while you're at it? Then maybe, there's a chance that the person you're in love with will pay attention and realize what they're missing.

But changing yourself is not the most reliable approach.

Imagine yourself actually succeeding with this radical makeover. You have newer cooler duds (expensive), behave differently (almost impossible) and your muscles are toned (long, boring hours at the gym). If you succeed in getting your crush interested in you this way, you've still failed. Connecting with someone when you have recreated yourself for them means you have set yourself up to play a role, which you then have to live up to. You'd have to practice really hard every waking moment to hide your real personality. Your heart's desire would be attracted to this person that you have forced yourself to be, not who you really are.

It's better to spend your time and energy trying to get to know the person you're interested in. In the end, it's pretty depressing to pair up with someone who cares more about what sneakers you wear than about your personality. You deserve to be loved and appreciated for who you are, not the person you're pretending to be, and so does everyone else. A relationship can't be based on an act.

Going Out

Yes! Yes! Yes! You're in a relationship. You're with someone. You're not used to not being single anymore yet. You're paired up. Going steady. Whoa. Maybe you know your boyfriend or girlfriend quite well already. Or maybe you're still basically strangers. An almost brand-new person for you to get to know, inside and out. The physical and mental exploration begins. In the best-case scenario, you accept the person's bad sides and revel in their good sides.

Next you start wondering about things. You're still so new to each other you can't find the courage yet to ask them the tough questions. For example – how long do we wait to have sex? Three weeks, three months or three years? You can't know in advance, and again, there is no rule that works for everyone. The only thing that's certain is that no one has the right to demand sex from you — and you can't demand it from another person, either. Since there are no laws against consensual sex between two minors or two adults, it's up to the two of you.

When you start hanging out with a new person (especially someone you're in love with) it can be hard to be yourself. Maybe you decide to play it cool and try not to be too "into it." You stop yourself from giving too many compliments and try to keep the number of phone calls to a minimum. Again, these methods usually don't work too well. A relationship will die if both people don't get affirmation and support. You and your partner need to hear how fantastic and gorgeous you both are. Plus it's pretty hard for him or her to get to know you if you're busy playing games and acting.

If you're new to relationships, it's tempting to think that reality is like the movies. Why don't we ever make out for five hours in a row on a park bench, or pour honey and whipped cream on each other in the middle of the night? This attitude is bound to leave you feeling disappointed. Overall, it's best not to spend too much time comparing. Every romantic relationship is unique and there is no authority that decides what a happy or successful relationship is like. For example, you might start imagining that you and your partner are in love in the same way. But that's often not the case. Love fluctuates. One week one person feels more and the next week, it's the other person. That doesn't have to be a bad thing — on the contrary, this common pattern can actually work like an engine that pushes the relationship along. The person who is the most in love struggles hard to preserve it. And sometimes, struggle can be a good thing. You might see the relationship with fresh eyes and stop taking things for granted.

Fighting

Sometimes I think the human race could be divided into two types of people: those who fight and those who avoid fighting. Often, a non-fighter ends up with a fighter, which can cause various complications. The non-fighter hides in the closet while the fighter stands outside sharpening his or her claws. The good news is that we can learn a lot from these relationships. The avoider can get better at confrontation, and the aggressive person can learn to calm down.

People often claim that it's good and healthy to clear the air and scream at each other a little. That does seem to work for some people. But constant arguments can also jeopardize the relationship.

Useful tips for the conflict avoider

There are plenty of advantages to being like you. As calm as a Buddhist monk, you walk around with a serene expression on your face. But there are drawbacks, too. Your fighter friends, girlfriends or boyfriends, can easily take advantage of you. Since they're skilled at arguing, they might be able to get you to apologize when you haven't done anything wrong. In the worst case scenario, you avoid bringing up problems because you're worried that she/he will start screaming. For these reasons you need find a way to bring up problems and point out hurts and mistakes. To get over your fear of confrontation, try to prepare yourself. Write down what you want to say. Choose whether to sit down with your partner face-to-face or write them a letter. The major advantage of a letter is that the criticized person can't start shouting defensive statements right away. Letters are slower and require more thought.

Useful tips for the fighter
You have a short fuse. The advantage of being you is that it's hard for others to abuse you. But many fighters have a hard time hearing criticism and often refuse to look inward to see if the criticism is merited.

If someone criticizes you, try to remain calm. Think carefully about whether the person has a point. Tell them what you agree with and what you think is unfair. Don't just stick to your side of the story. Remember that in a relationship, a fight is not a competition — if your partner loses, in a way you've lost, too.

Breaking Up
Breaking up can be one of the hardest things in the world. But even though it's tough, sad and scary, it's something you're probably going to have to go through. When two people start going out, both of them risk getting hurt and hurting the other person. The risk that it will end is part of the nature of a relationship. Besides the difficult task of breaking up, it can be awful to deal with the feeling that the end is coming. One sign is if kissing feels more like a chore than a pleasure. If spotting your boyfriend or girlfriend doesn't excite you, or if you keep making excuses or half-lies to get out of seeing them, those are sure signs, too. Living in a relationship that has died isn't good for anyone. Better to take the bull by the horns and find the courage to face the issue.

But how will she/he react? With tears, anger or quiet sadness? Maybe it's best to just go on an extended trip to another country, or move to a remote mountaintop? Tempting fantasy, I know. But you do actually owe the person you were once infatuated with some basic respect. They have a right to look into your eyes when you tell them it's over, and you need to let them ask questions. You're smart enough to figure out which break-up methods are just plain wrong. Getting a friend to do it, sending a text message or simply avoiding the person are just a few examples. Just because you can steer clear of the person's sorrow doesn't mean that they aren't feeling it.

Preparing for the break-up will make it a bit easier. The most important thing is that you tell the person why you're breaking up. You should stick to the truth as much as possible. Claiming that you have to move on because you need more time to study when you've both got the same exams is just insulting. But here's the tricky part: don't be too honest, either. You don't need to let her or him know that you didn't like the way she/he babbled constantly or that she/he had bad breath or that you fantasize about your best friend when you jerk off. Keep the hurtful details to yourself.

Once you've broken up with the person, you should avoid making out or having sex with them. Plenty of people have made the mistake of having sex "as friends" after a break-up, but unless you want to be remembered as a user and a liar, it's a really dumb idea. Keep your hands to yourself and do the best you can to respond to the dumpee's questions. Doing anything else is beneath you. Afterward, you'll feel like a massive weight has been lifted from your shoulders and you'll have grown as a person. Sure, your ex might feel sad or even miserable, but you can't change that.

Getting Dumped

One day it's over. The person you're crazy about has ended it. You've been dumped. Down in the dumps, thrown out to the curb with all the other rejected and abandoned people. New questions come up all the time. What's wrong with me? What did I do wrong? Am I ever going to feel loved again? The days flow together, everything feels wrong, and all the while, your loved one is drifting further and further away. There's no one to ask why it's all over.

What we often forget in this situation is that this isn't the end of your entire love life. I can guarantee that you will fall in love again. It's a cliché, but it's true: there are lots of fish in the sea. When the worst grief is over, a new, happy world almost always opens up again.

Getting dumped can feel like a letdown and a failure. Telling your friends and family about it can be really challenging, because you've temporarily forgotten what everyone else knows: everyone gets dumped sometime. There's no shame in getting dumped.

You might feel like taking revenge on the dumper. Maybe you spread rumors or reveal secrets. But that's going to tarnish the whole relationship, like desecrating a grave. It's undignified. Try to remember that breaking up is not a crime. Don't ruin all the memories of the great moments that you likely did share. I can't think of a single situation when vengeance would be an effective remedy for the sadness dumpees usually feel. And often, it's the person who is bent on payback that everyone sees as being in the wrong. The best revenge is no revenge at all. Setting aside childish behavior and moving on is the best thing you can do for yourself.

Another common feeling when you get dumped is that you're shrinking or almost disappearing. Your self-esteem has received a bad blow, and it's hard to smile at yourself in the mirror. Just try hard to banish negative thinking from your mind. Before long, your confidence will be on the mend.

What's your advice for someone who has just been dumped?

Mike, 16
Getting dissed by a girl in front of all your friends is brutally embarrassing because they all make fun of you. But whatever. It

might have nothing to do with anything you did. It could be you were with the wrong girl and it wasn't meant to be.

Lisa, 17

It's incredibly painful. You don't know where to turn at first, but it does get better. It sounds like the world's biggest cliché but it's true. Try to think about other things, hang out with people who make you happy, and talk to a counselor if you need to. If it feels right, you can keep in contact with your ex, but usually it's really hard because you're reminded of everything all the time. Even if it's tough, you'll probably feel better if you break contact with the person.

Christina, 16

Try to hang out with friends… Tell yourself that it was her/his loss and that you'll find someone who appreciates and deserves you.

Stuart, 16

I talked about this with a friend and she thought you should try to start hating the person who dumped you. I think it's the opposite. You should be happy about the good times you had with the person. But try not to fall into a pit of despair, and get on with your life as fast as you can. Maybe you can try to find someone new. It's also important to take time for yourself and be a bit selfish.

I Don't Want to Fall in Love

Sometimes it can feel like everyone talks about love. Tight-knit couples line the halls at school. As soon as you flick on the TV, there's some couple making eyes at each other, and when your parents get home they ask if there's a cute girl you like at school. It can be a pain having to tell people for the umpteenth time that no, you haven't met anyone special and you don't even want to meet anyone. Most people want to find someone to be with, so they often forget that it doesn't apply to everyone. So many situations in our society revolve around love and coupledom. Movies, books, even video games. In the end it can feel like there's some obscure punishment in store for the weirdo who doesn't go mushy over anyone. But there isn't. Everyone has the right not to be interested in anyone. You can feel and experience love as much — or as little — as you want.

Jealousy

They're everywhere you look. People with dark, bitter expressions and gritted teeth. Jealousy is very common, and it can feel like you're condemned to resent your partner, your ex, the person you love who doesn't love you back, and so on.

Feeling jealous now and again is normal, but in larger doses it's harmful and unhealthy. Jealousy makes a lot of people try to control their partners, which can turn the relationship into a dictatorship. Imagine you start going out with an amazing, cool person. At the start, everything's great. But after just a few weeks, issues start coming up. Your partner isn't too psyched when you go out to meet your close circle of friends. When you see the person next, she/he questions you about it. You realize that the person you're with doesn't want you to hang out with other people at all, because every time the questions are more detailed and paranoid. Whenever you see each other, the conversations are all about what you do when you're not together. Your love interest might threaten to break up if you keep meeting up with someone they're worried about. Above all, if you're straight, you're not allowed to hang out with people of the opposite sex.

Lots of people live this way — with lovers who try to own them. This starts to feel like you're having a relationship with a cop or a prison warden — neither pleasant nor romantic. Being together doesn't mean you have a right to decide who the other person should and should not spend time with. And being in a couple doesn't mean you should have to give up your own friends and interests. On the contrary, it's essential that you both keep your own lives going.

When your girlfriend or boyfriend starts interrogating you and throwing their suspicions and fears in your face, think carefully about how to react. The risk is that you are so desperate to make up that you placate them in order to make everything OK. But bending to their will and promising to change (when you've done nothing wrong) means saying goodbye to fairness in your relationship. Instead, try initiating a talk where you explain that you have a right to see your friends.

Jealousy is kind of an unnecessary feeling, but we're all troubled by it at some point. Jealousy can make you imagine strange things. Like, for example, that your girlfriend is making out with Tom in the library when really they're just studying for a math test together. If you're being affected by dark, paranoid feelings about your partner, try to calm down and think about what you're feeling and why. Don't forbid your girlfriend to see Tom, or anyone else. She's an independent person and you don't want her to fail her math test. Think instead about what these jealous feelings say about you. Jealousy can be rooted in your own self-esteem issues. If you feel you have to force this person to stick around, maybe it's because you don't believe they will stick around of their own free will.

Being waylaid by feelings of jealousy hurts both you and the person you're going out with. So what do you do with the feelings, and how do you find out what's really going on? Go to Tom's house one night and just let him have it? Start spying through the library windows? Go through your girlfriend's pockets for evidence of wrongdoing? You got it — none of these ideas are sane or reasonable.

Instead of skulking around, just bite the bullet and initiate a conversation about the feelings and fears you are having. Ask the person to help you look inward. If you can bring yourself to admit that you feel insecure, sad or hurt about something else in your life, you will probably both feel better and closer afterwards. Remember that the jealousy is clouding your perspective, making it harder to see the truth.

Chapter 5
Equality

Equality: A state of being essentially equal or equivalent; equally balanced.

In ninth grade I started seeing things differently than I had before. I wondered why guys and girls are the way they are. Suddenly it felt like masculinity and femininity were a bit scary and hard to live up to. I felt like we might lose something important on the way to figuring out who we were as men and women.

I was even a bit envious of the girls: they seemed to be able to talk to each other about their feelings. We guys were different. You couldn't appear weak or admit you were wrong; instead, you had to work really hard to cover up your flaws. We had to be tough all the time and pump ourselves up to each other, so talking about problems when we were hanging out just didn't work. It felt like being earnest or vulnerable just wasn't allowed. When we talked about sex, we had to pretend we knew everything. We acted like we were experienced.

But although the guys' world felt harsh and ruthless at times, there was stuff about the girls' world that I was glad I didn't have to deal with. In some classes, girls seemed to talk less, not because they had less to say, but because the guys talked so much there was no time left. Girls were more easily exposed to rumors. If they dressed ultra-sexy or went out with several different guys, they'd be called sluts. But they were still expected to keep their bodies trim and look hot all the time, especially if they wanted to avoid being called dogs or lesbos. They had to walk a fine line, that's for sure. What's more, it seemed like some guys saw the girls as just a nice body or a great face. Sometimes this view seemed to rub off on the girls, so they would start seeing themselves as a pair of great legs, a slim waist – or a fat ass or flat chest.

If we made out or had sex with a lot of people (or claimed we did), we were called players or studs. This was usually a good thing. How come there were such different rules for girls and guys?

The more I thought about it, the more I realized there had always been one set of rules for guys and another for girls. Some of the rules may have changed a bit since kindergarten, but even then, most boys had learned to avoid being soft or needy. We were encouraged to wrestle and play sports, to be little men who pretended to be tough and didn't cry when we got hurt. Everything was a competition to decide who was a sissy. Some teachers expected us to be wild in the schoolyard during breaks, whereas the girls were subtly told to be calmer and better behaved. I would rather have taken it easy and explored things by myself or with the girls, but I remember feeling that it wasn't completely acceptable and would probably have gotten me kicked out of the cool crowd. And as a little kid, all I wanted to do was to fit in.

Not that I thought about any of this back then. But I had a feeling of not exactly fitting in or being allowed to be the person I actually was. The male world was for tough guys, and that world was perpetuated throughout grade school.

By the time I made it to high school, I started to get how much both girls and guys were losing out because of this rigid framework of rules. In their quest for "masculinity," guys were forced to get rid of qualities that didn't fit, and the same was true for girls with their "femininity." A bunch of my best traits were considered "effeminate." It took me a long time, but eventually I stopped pretending and trying to hide those parts of myself, and soon I felt way better.

The Slut and Sissy System

At school there are other demands besides studying, test scores and grades. There is another whole set of requirements that doesn't come from parents or teachers. Your friends and classmates place demands on you. There are unwritten rules that decide how you act, how you dress – and how you absolutely should not dress or act.

There's a system that controls many of our society's young peer groups which ensures that members stick to accepted behaviors. I call it the slut and sissy system. A girl can't be too bold and she can't seek open sexual enjoyment from whomever she wants. If she gets close to "too many" or "too sexy" territory, she's labeled something like "slut." This doesn't necessarily mean that she's had sex with anyone — she could simply be interested in several people, be too frank or forward, or wear a shirt that shows her belly-button.

A guy should be strong and tough. He can't be too nice or too good at expressing what he feels. He is encouraged to be physically accomplished, and is respected if he "scores" make-out sessions with lots of girls. And he absolutely can't be interested in screwing around with other guys. If a guy fails on any of these counts, he's labeled something like "sissy."

This system of rules eats away at our individual freedom. If any person or group dictates how you ought to act, dress or make out, it limits your development as a person. Chances are you might paint yourself into a mental corner as you obsess over how to fit all the regulations.

The rules say that girls are one way and guys another. Why?

Does a girl have to be more empathetic, nurturing and attractive, but less daring? Does a guy have to be more competitive, have thicker skin and be less capable of talking about how he feels? The answer is no. Who or what decides that it should be this way? Nature? Hardly.

The term "gender role" often comes up in discussions about equality. Before the twentieth century, our society was built around distinct roles for thousands of years: women played one role and men played another. These roles really had next to nothing to do with nature or biology, nor had the roles always been the same before our civilization. This makes me so mad. A lot of guys need to talk about their feelings and love to nurture plants and animals. Shouldn't they be able to do what they want to do? Should a girl have to hide her oil-stained hands if she's into building go-karts? The reality is that if you accept these gender roles, you face the prospect of having to cut off parts of your own personality. Being a guy doesn't mean just being interested in typical male things. It sounds corny, but I'll say it: instead of fitting in, focus on being yourself. Thankfully, everyone has parts of their personality that are outside of these limited gender roles, and often they can be the most cool and unique parts.

The gender system isn't just built by you and your peer group. There are people painting your personality into a corner all over the place: daycare workers, teachers, parents, coaches, doctors... You learn a lot about gender roles at home, too, so the rules get enforced very early on. Be careful who you let whisper in your ear: whenever someone says, "Toughen up," calls you a sissy, or otherwise tells you what a man is supposed to be like, an alarm should go off inside you. Remind yourself that you get to decide what a guy – a guy like you – is like.

You're Not Born a Man

When I was nearing the end of grade school, our class went on a weekend camping trip. Our days were packed with activity. We went on excursions, collecting samples of animal and plant species. Besides our homeroom teacher, some parents came with us, including one kid's dad. He got to take the boys around and do typical guy things with us. We skipped rocks, wrestled and raced. But mostly, we listened to his stories. They were about picking up women, playing the casinos and getting drunk with his buddies. He loved to tell us that, from his own big success with women, it was clear that most women liked "real men" – men like him. He also told us how one day he demolished an armchair because he'd been so enraged when he got home and realized his wife had left the liquor cabinet empty. He'd let the "old lady" know what was what, he said proudly. She was obsessed with "stupid woman stuff," as he called it, like the house and cooking – we men, he said, were more interested in really living, like going to the game and tying one on.

I met a few other men like this around the same time. They were coaches, friends' fathers and substitute teachers – and somehow, they all wanted to set an example for my friends and me by talking about sex, booze and sports, and by trashing women and homosexuals. Looking back, I realize these men scared me a little, but at the same time, their stories were fascinating to listen to. I thought they were handing down the True Gospel of Adulthood. Sometimes I would try to act like these bigheaded, boastful men. Often I couldn't pull it off, but now and then I'd be rewarded with awed or impressed looks from my posse when I spat on the sidewalk or screamed "pussy" at some scared little guy in the schoolyard.

In 1949, author and philosopher Simone de Beauvoir wrote in her famous feminist work *The Second Sex* that "One is not born a woman. One becomes a woman." I think she's dead on, and the same thing goes for guys. We're not born men. We become men. Often in quite painful ways, through struggles, disappointments, blood and sweat.

I learned what is male from, among other sources, the big-headed men who seemed to be everywhere when I was growing up. Somehow I learned to admire men for their piggish behavior. Really, it wasn't much to look up to. And I realize now that they probably didn't quite know how to be men. In most situations, it's inappropriate to talk about trashing armchairs. Maybe that's why these men were spreading their rotten values to us when we weren't even in our teens yet. We listened and didn't question; we just sat there with shiny eyes, taking it all in.

There is No Power Tool Gene

Time and again you'll encounter opinions about how men and women have always been some specific way. Nature and biology dictate it, these believers claim. Women should be at home with the kids and men should bring home the bacon. These attitudes are not just held by random individuals; there is actually a lot of research on this topic. Researchers working in this field actively seek evidence that men and women work differently. Often the studies are very strange. A classic variant is to test a group of women against a group of men. And, as you might expect, one group always wins. The fact is, no matter which two groups you set up against each other — imagine the hipsters against the home-boys at your high school — one group always wins.

Besides, these studies have an even more basic weakness: the people being tested are shaped by the society we all live in. If you do a study to prove that men are better at using power tools than women, you'll be proving what you already know to be true: that boys are more often encouraged and taught to use power tools than girls. What it doesn't prove is that boys are born with something like a power tool gene.

Another common research method is to measure and study the brain in the hopes of finding differences between groups of people. We've been doing this for over a century in the Western world, and the practice reached its most repulsive phase in Hitler's Germany, when Nazi doctors tried to find biological evidence for the superiority of the Aryan race. Obviously, that particular area of study is no longer taken seriously, but using this method to understand how men and women differ still seems to be acceptable. Usually, scientists don't do these studies out of the goodness of their hearts: someone with ulterior motives is paying for proof that men are inherently different from women. And in the end, it's not very challenging to point out differences if you're looking for them.

One thing's for sure: you'll be exposed to tons of study results that conflict with each other. Read the newspaper two weekends in a row and you'll see what I mean. The words "research" and "evidence" sound weighty. But the next time you read something like "New study proves that women are better at housecleaning than men," or "Researchers find the male gene responsible for superior cognitive abilities," be very suspicious. Yes, it's true that women often clean house better than men, but that has nothing to do with nature or biology. Keep in mind that if someone "proves" that men are more capable than women, they're not the first. The inferiority of women has been "verified" many times over the past centuries, but in the end, the research methods of these studies have always been proven inaccurate.

If you're prepared to accept shoddy evidence, there are plenty of studies proving differences between the sexes. But if you want the truth, and real proof to go along with it, you'll have a much tougher time. One distinction is plain to the naked eye: women have breasts and a vagina, whereas men have a penis. Leave it at that, and remember the most important fact of all: differences between individuals — whether female or male — are much more plentiful and significant than those between the genders.

Our ideals and expectations of gender are not written in stone, nor is it God or nature that decides what is male or female. Even supposing they did, the huge variation in human gender roles and behavior would certainly give you the impression that both God and nature are comfortable with uncertainty.

It is intuitively obvious that car mechanics and power tools haven't always been part of what is considered male. Having a penis doesn't make someone long for race cars or guns. Masculinity and femininity have always changed and will continue to do so — and that's why we all have an opportunity to have an effect on what we think is wrong or bad about the way things are today.

Macho Man vs Modern Man

Fashion and beauty ideals have often made people do stupid things. How smart is it to wear a corset so tight that you faint all the time and can't eat? The same goes for the male role. Think of it as a straitjacket or a controlling parent: they keep you from being the real you.

Take the old saying, "like a bull in a china shop." Everyone knows that china shop owners aren't thrilled by visits from bulls. But it's probably even worse for the bull: it feels awkward and clumsy. The bull might try to control himself but he just can't. The bull is too inflexible. The macho man is the same way. He is hard and clumsy. Macho will work sometimes, but far from always. In love relationships and in many other contexts, the macho man is a bull who can't maneuver his way around other people.

The macho guy sees masculinity as something superior and he doesn't give feelings a lot of credit. He has never learned to share his feelings with anyone, so he is a kind of pressure cooker. To feel good as a person, you have to relieve the pressure. But the macho man hasn't found his vent. So, quite often, he explodes.

Love and relationships scare most macho men because to love you have to expose yourself. They believe that exposing themselves to feelings puts them at too much risk for failure. And macho men must not fail.

The crisis of masculinity has been a popular topic of discussion for the last couple of decades. A bunch of theorists have claimed that men are losing their identity because, for the first time, we are in an age where men are no longer irreplaceable. Nowadays there are barely any tasks that only men are equipped for. And to purist macho men, this turn of events makes them feel powerless and gives rise to a strong backlash reaction.

During the 1990s, a men's movement sprung up that centered on the search for a new, better, healthier masculinity. For the most part, this movement builds on the ideals of equality that the women's movements brought forward during the 1960s, 1970s and 1980s. This model of masculinity sees men as taking part in child rearing and treating their partners as equals. This men's movement joins forces with the women's movement in organizing against issues of inequality between the sexes, such as fighting violence against women, or extending parental leave to men.

There is another part of the men's movement that has different goals. Some men read the book *Iron John* by Robert Bly and have turned back to old versions of manhood as they supposedly existed in pre-modern eras. *Iron John* presents some odd ideas. Among other things, it claims that boys become men by doing typically "male" things with adult men. When the boy learns to use a bow and arrow or fish, a mysterious substance is transferred from the older man to the younger boy, and he becomes a man. Bly's ideas have been criticized as being too mystical.

Then there's the worst part of the men's movement, which

wants to fight against equality and the women's movements that have fought for it. These groups insist that men are worse off than women because women's achievements in equality have gone too far. But when you listen carefully to these views, you can hear a self-pitying aspiration to turn back the clock and return to the past, when men's power wasn't questioned.

Of course, it's good that we try to understand how men's roles have changed and what the consequences are for guys who are growing up now. But what's scary about the anti-feminist men's movement, or the family values movement as it is also called in the United States, is that it focuses on the plight and strengths of only the male gender. Even worse, it often leads to a vengeful, backward-looking mindset. Another major risk of this approach is that the men's movement tries to create one definition of manhood. We need lots of definitions of manhood. One for every man, in fact.

The modern man doesn't allow himself to be limited by long-gone ideals or the judgmental gaze of outsiders. He is who he wants to be, and he does the things he wants to do even if they're not considered "manly." This gives him the freedom to become a great cook and ride a motorcycle, or hug his best friend and learn to box. Since he allows himself to be touched and have feelings, he can experience love and have great sex.

It takes strength and courage to be a modern man, especially in high school. There are plenty of people on hand to dish out all the typical insults — but if you develop the confidence to be yourself, you'll learn to expect these attempts to slander your image, and you'll stop caring.

There is lots of tricky stuff to deal with in high school. Male friendship is one of them. Guy friends are supposed to be tough and kind of sarcastic toward each other. You'll be pushed to avoid being empathetic or sensitive. That weird backslapping routine is fine, but hugging or otherwise expressing affection is out. Even though some girls confess to being sick of the cozy sleepover makeover parties, that kind of togetherness just seems healthier than the bruiser games that guys use to get close.

Personally, I gradually stopped seeing the "softer" parts of myself as a handicap. I became more and more self-assured and refused to let myself be limited by macho culture. Soon, I noticed other guys like me in the community starting to come out of the woodwork. It was such an epiphany when I realized there are loads of guys who don't fight, boast or try to win all the time.

I believe the modern man stands up to the macho man any day. Not that it's a competition.

Collective Responsibility and Guilt

Sometimes I'll end up behind a girl when I'm walking home alone at night. I can tell from her body language that she's on guard. I wonder how I can show from a distance that I'm harmless. What does a harmless person look like? She turns around apprehensively quite a few times. I want to call out, "Not all guys have violent tendencies!"

Chances are that you too will frighten lots of people even though you're a complete stranger to them — just by walking down the street. That might feel really unfair — what have you done to make them fear you? But it's no wonder, given how common it is for women of all ages to experience sexual violence in their lives — whether at home in private, or out in public. So how do you deal with the conflicting reality that there are lots of violent men, but you're not one of them?

Think about the difference between guilt and responsibility. All guys should not have to feel guilty because there are men who humiliate, assault and rape. We are not to blame for having a penis. On the other hand, we should all feel collectively responsible. You might have experienced this feeling of responsibility when you noticed that a woman was afraid of you because you're a guy. For this reason, it's our duty to show that we are not threatening or sleazy. If someone has a biased opinion about you, it's up to you to prove the person wrong. The most important thing is awareness. Be conscious of the fact that girls can be intimidated, and ask what you can do about it. Take a stand if you see someone being sexually harassed. Speak your mind if someone starts spouting crappy views about women or brings old sexist jokes out of the closet where they belong.

I have to admit that I'm not great at that sort of thing. If I see someone actually being physically harassed I take action. But I have a really hard time saying something when a guy spews contempt for women in the change room. (Maybe that's why I'm writing this book instead.)

If you're like me, you do have some alternatives. Train yourself to muster up the courage to make your opinion heard. At least, learn not to just sit there and agree with other guys' rotten opinions. The loudest guy might call you an idiot, but the other guys sitting silent will probably be relieved that someone is saying something that makes sense for a change.

You could also go straight to the girl in question to show that you are aware of the situation she is in, and that you are prepared to back her up if she takes action. Believe me, it can mean a lot to her.

When a girl faces sexual harassment or assault, it's common that she starts to doubt herself and the guys around her. She may even convince herself that the situation isn't that bad. By talking to her, you show that there are good guys around, and that someone takes her situation seriously. She might believe that what she's going through isn't serious enough to bring up with the administration, she may fear the consequences of getting the guy in trouble, or she may have already told them, to no avail. You can acknowledge the reality of her situation and support her in doing what's right to address it. Ask her if she wants you to go with her to talk to the principal. I can guarantee that she needs support from someone, so why not you?

You can always go right to the source: talk to the guy. Tell him you know what he's doing and that you don't approve. Even if he's the toughest guy in the school, somewhere inside, he'll be scared half to death. If you can't face talking to him yourself, get one of your more gutsy friends to do it. Or write him an anonymous note.

Some people might think it sounds weird to go around putting things right after other guys have behaved badly. But it's not. We don't just help the girls who are affected but also ourselves. We counteract the fear that women and girls can feel when they see a man on a deserted street, and the preconceived notions that people have about men. If enough guys take a stand, the public won't be able to lump all men into one group, and fewer women will be exposed. It's up to each one of us.

Feminism

They don't want to destroy you and they don't hate men. The feminist movement has improved conditions for many women and men over the last few decades. And yet, lots of people prefer to focus on the negatives rather than the positives. Feminists are labeled man-haters and ball-busters rather than heroes. It's as if there's a contest for who can come up with the most derogatory thing to say about feminists. "They destroy the fabric of the family" or "they are fanatics" and "they harp on problems that no longer exist" — these are all statements that I have heard from guys my age. No one would talk this way about men who took up a political fight, but when it comes to women's political issues, it seems totally acceptable to throw around rude, aggressive comments. It's not just men who participate in putting down feminists: lots of women take part in the mud-slinging, too. "They're trying to tell me that there is a problem with who I am," they say. The opposite is actually true: feminism today takes into account all sorts of women. In fact, feminism is about breaking apart gender stereotypes. Feminists are freedom fighters.

Of course, there are lots of different movements and groups that call themselves feminist. Some of them are the more radical kind, while others are simply about breaking down the walls between the genders. A few feminists here and there are angry and want to distance themselves from men, but in general, feminism has achieved huge positive change for both women and men.

The basic definition of feminism is to fight for equal rights between men and women, and for the eradication of women's second-rate status. So I figure, given this description, it would be weird if I didn't consider myself a feminist. It's a politically charged word that has strong feelings attached to it, so many people make a face when I talk about my acceptance of feminism. I've had people ask me how a man can be a feminist. Doesn't the word itself make that impossible? Of course not. Should I not care about the issue of equality just because it was first addressed by the women's movement? Maybe it's just me, but it's pretty obvious that if my girlfriend has fewer rights than I have, we're both worse off. So I figure that we modern men should see it as our right and our duty to care about the cause of equal rights — we should take every opportunity we can to speak out against unfairness and to tell others about our ideas and ideals.

After early women's movements secured the woman's right to vote in the early part of the twentieth century, the feminist movement broke through in a really big way in the US during the Swinging Sixties. Soon, it spread throughout the Western world. Feminists invented a bunch of new concepts that have had a huge effect on how women and men in the West see themselves. A lot of people now agree that women and men are shaped by the societal possibilities around us rather than by the biological tools we are born with.

Another thing the feminists have made us see is that somehow, men are taken as the norm. The theory, originating with Simone de Beauvoir, goes something like this: since men usually occupy the positions of power, men write our books, which essentially means they are writing our history and memory, and therefore our frames of reference. So man has become the norm, while woman is "the other." Think about it: it's still easy to find thousands of everyday examples of this phenomenon. Turn on the television, and notice how the announcers talk about the NHL and the Women's Hockey League. We don't say the "Men's Hockey League:" it's enough to just say NHL hockey. Because men's hockey is "normal" hockey. And think about what mankind means: humankind. Saying mankind doesn't mean you're referring to just people with penises.

The person who is the norm doesn't see himself that way. The white middle class man who looks himself in the mirror just sees a person; while a person who is not the norm – like a woman or a black man – feels more defined by being a woman or being black. What's my point here? Sometimes it's hard for men, maybe especially white men, to notice the unfairness. But women still make less money than men for the same job, and men still occupy 90 percent of the top ranks of all the major corporations in the Western world.

But I Don't Want to Lose My Power

There are men who are worried about equality because they don't want to give up any of their own power. They want to keep all the benefits of being a man intact and wonder what equality will mean on a practical level. Questions like, "Would I have to serve the women in my life, give up my job, or have my butt pinched?" sound ridiculous, but some men really do have it all backwards. Equality is not about women taking over men's roles. It means ensuring that all women and men will be seen simply as individuals, each with their own characteristics and qualities. Men would in all likelihood enjoy more success at work if all jobs were filled with the most competent person, female or male.

As I mentioned, it makes the most sense to think of equality as a win-win situation. If we could get rid of the worst aspects of both the male and the female roles in society, we would all be better off. When men and women get stuck on either side of the so-called war of the sexes, it is as if they speak two different languages. We all need some perspective: the walls that divide us are walls that we created in the first place, and the last thing the world needs is another soldier defending these artificial barriers. So don't get stuck being a foot soldier for the male side of an old battle that should no longer be fought.

Girls Who Seek Out Tough Guys

Some girls are drawn to tough guys. The kind of guys you always hear and see more of than anybody else. When you look out at the schoolyard and see the tough guy surrounded by a bunch of pretty girls, it's impossible not to feel a twinge of envy or even anger. Why do they want him? He lies, gets drunk, fights and treats girls like crap. Next, you might think, "I should forget about this whole nice-guy routine, since nasty hardcore guys get all the girls."

But I don't buy that. Even if you make up a mean, evil-guy act, how would you treat your would-be girlfriend? Give her the cold shoulder one minute and grab her ass the next? Tell her she shouldn't bother with all this school stuff since girls are only good for one thing? Forget it. Being yourself is just easier. And at least then there's still a chance that someone will fall for who you really are.

Violence

I'm on my way to the subway. And it hits me that it's not just girls and women who are afraid of aggressive or intimidating men. The girl in front of me tenses up when she hears my steps, but I'm a little nervous, too.

Who is walking behind me? And what if the person is dangerous? I turn around. No one is there. After this major street, I tell myself, there is a mall with lots of people, and the voice in my head will subside. Being scared and showing it can feel humiliating. Who am I scared of? What am I scared of? Who has a right to frighten me? During the day, I feel fine in the streets; I move and dress however I want to. But at night, in specific environments, it's different. The fear keeps me from going everywhere I want to go and forces me to be aware of potential threats. A big guy with a grim face gives me a long look as he passes me, and I feel myself hunching over. Someone has gotten enjoyment out of scaring me. I realize it has made me mad: what makes someone want to frighten and maybe even assault another person? Is there anyone who likes to be scared? OK, maybe on a winter night in front of a horror movie with a bowl of popcorn, or safely in my own bedroom with a playful blindfold – but not by a stranger, and not when I haven't given my explicit consent.

Somehow, things are out of whack in our society. Most humans are caught in a spiral of fear and aggression, particularly those of us who live in big cities. This guy with the big boots on my left: is he belligerent? Or maybe he's scared of me for some reason, too. Chances are that neither of us has any reason to fear each other. But some people do stand to gain within this circle of fear and violence: the toughest, most spiteful people. It's easy to see that, under this system, the wrong people win.

A Manifesto – Sort of

All of us have the amazing freedom to make change happen. By daring to be ourselves we can also change others. We don't have to be like our fathers, and we have the right to ignore the invisible rules about what "manly" behavior is — those rules belong in the past. None of us can do it alone, but the more aware we are of how we want the world to look, the easier it is to act in accordance with our own vision.

We should enable each other to get out of the spiral of fear and violence. My contribution is to remind you, my readers, how much we all stand to gain by dropping the aggressive approach and the tendency toward violence. My pledge is to avoid being provoked, and to behave in a non-threatening way.

We should strive to find injustice and point it out to others without feeling awkward. When someone tells you that you have to be a certain way because that's how boys are, show them that the opposite is true: no one knows you better than you know yourself. Just because we might have seen sexism, racism and homophobia in our teachers, coaches or parents, doesn't mean that we need to adopt those values. Instead, take advantage of your youth status and do and say what others don't expect.

We don't slap asses, call people "fags" or swing our fists around when we get frustrated. When we say we deserve respect, it doesn't mean that we want others to fear us and our buddies when we walk down the street. It simply means that they should take us at face value. And we give others the same respect. We listen, but we also feel comfortable disagreeing with others. We give everyone a chance and don't judge until we have gotten to know someone. Being surprised by people is something we cherish: it feels good to question and change our own views and opinions. Because, like everyone, we have biases, too — but we do our best to become aware and rise above them.

We can have a freedom that our parents and our parents' parents didn't have. The most free and honorable generation yet. It starts with us and we know that if we grab our freedom, others will follow. We don't steal our freedom from others: we create more freedom for everyone by being who we want to be. It's a fun and important job. And if we haven't done it yet, we can start now.

Chapter 6
Gay

What do Greg Louganis, Elton John and Cary Grant have in common with guys like Plato, Oscar Wilde, Shakespeare and Michelangelo? Answer: All of them are, or were, gay or bisexual. Oscar Wilde, who lived during the last half of the 1800s, suffered pretty serious persecution for his homosexuality. Despite being a hugely popular author and playwright, he was sent to prison because of his sexual preference. For the Greek philosopher Plato, who lived from 427 to 348 BC, the situation was very different. In ancient Greece, sexual relations between men were considered the best and most pure type of human love. People believed that love between men was "manlier" than love between a man and a woman. Male bodies were worshipped, and songs and poems about beautiful young men were everywhere. Plato could engage exclusively in same-sex sexual activities without raising any eyebrows at all.

The concept of homosexuality wasn't invented until the 1800s. Everywhere the concept took root, people started identifying and trying to "cure" gay people instead of punishing them. Homosexuality was seen as a disease and no longer as a mortal sin, as it had been during the first fifteen centuries of Christianity. To some degree, it was a step forward that gays were no longer condemned to punishments like stoning — but the "treatments" were cruel and gays often died during their "therapy."

In the early 1900s, a rich and varied gay culture was established in Berlin. There were more than a hundred bars and clubs for gays, and even specialized services, like detective and employment agencies. A community paper, *Die Freundschaft* (*The Friendship*), was by the late 1920s published in 100,000-copy print runs. In 1922, four hundred people convened in Berlin for the world's first demonstration opposing discrimination against gays and for the legalization of homosexuality.

But when the Nazis came to power in Germany in 1933, they quickly put a stop to the freedom and tolerance gays had enjoyed. Gay men were hunted down and sent to concentration camps or forced to wear pink triangles on their clothes to make their sexual preferences public. And even during the postwar period, when the Allies distributed reparation payments to groups persecuted by the Nazis, gay people were excluded because they continued to be despised.

A major reason that many cultures are so intolerant of homosexuality is because they have a restricted view of sex. Sex is for making babies, not for pleasure, according to this common view. So because gay sex is for pleasure, not reproduction, it has often been labeled as taboo or sinful.

In Canada, laws against gay male sex acts — referred to as "sodomy" — were repealed during the 1960s. And although the last anti-gay sex laws weren't repealed in all American states until 2003, a major turning point occurred in 1973 when homosexuality was eliminated as a disease from the DSM – the Diagnostic and Statistical Manual of Mental Disorders.

When the HIV/AIDS crisis started to spread in the mid-1980s, gay men again found themselves targets for reactionary forces in society who believed that HIV was sent by God as punishment for gays. (Although HIV first hit the news in 1981, scientists coined the term AIDS in 1982, and HIV was identified in 1983, it didn't really receive widespread media coverage until

Rock Hudson came out in 1985.) Attitudes toward and rights for gay people improved significantly in most Western countries during the 1990s and the early twenty-first century. The first same-sex marriage was made legal in the Netherlands in 2001. Gay and lesbian people are also free to marry in Belgium, Canada, South Africa, Spain and in one American state (Massachusetts). Canada is the only country where same-sex marriage has the same legal status as opposite-sex marriage. But there are still plenty of forces that make the lives of gays, bisexuals and transsexual and transgender people difficult.

Homophobia

It shouldn't matter who you fall in love with or who you think about when you masturbate. You ought to be allowed to shape your own sexuality and be whoever you want without being hassled. It shouldn't matter whether you make out with a girl or a guy. But there are plenty of things that people haven't gotten over yet, so things are not as self-evident as they ought to be.

There are people everywhere who just can't stop themselves from putting down others. People who make the world a crappier place by yelling "faggot" in the hallways, by making casual derogatory comments on the street or in private conversations. They might express disgust about gay sex, or they might describe straight relationships as more "real" or "authentic" than homosexual ones. Basically, there are a whole lot of folks who can't deal with the fact that not everyone is just like them. Homophobes try to make homosexuality into something that's ugly and repulsive. They can be your school buddies, your neighbors or your parents. Homophobes are everywhere: at school, in the police force, at camp or where you work.

I think homophobes are often afraid that they might be gay themselves. Maybe when they're trashing gays, they're really beating up that part of themselves. The school's toughest guy who's always repeating his latest "faggot" joke might lie awake at night wondering if he's gay. He's so afraid of being different that he starts to hate the little piece of himself that might be turned on by guys. Suddenly, it's not just the little piece of himself he hates, it's all gay people and homosexuality in general. By joking about bashing fags, he's trying to tell the world, "I'm not a fag."

Encountering an anti-gay bigot can be scary or nerve-wracking. But try not to let yourself be intimidated. Bigots can't get away with demoralizing others with their ignorance and stupidity. Try not to worry about being called a "faggot" by someone like that. Don't adjust to his or her version of reality. Accommodating homophobes means letting them win. So insist on being yourself in the face of homophobia: not just for your own self-esteem, but also as a crucial political act.

Lots of homophobes believe they are defending manhood, but they have a skewed idea of what being a man means. They somehow figure that the words "fag" and "man" are opposites. In their eyes, a man is someone who is attracted to women, but who is not a woman. And in their world, a "fag" is like a woman because he chooses a woman's — that is, the wrong — sex partner. So the gay man is not a "real" man. Lots of homophobes are afraid of being "unmanly." So they often take a tough guy's attitude toward both women and gays. Girls are for screwing, they seem to reason. But they forget that being a man has nothing to do with who you're screwing or who you're in love with.

What Causes Homosexuality?

If you're wondering why some people are gay and others are straight, you're not alone. Researchers, doctors and priests have tried to understand it for a long time. There have been plenty of theories. Homosexuality has been explained as a disease, a genetic predisposition, a socially learned behavior, a misguided choice and everything in between. But explanations or causes have often led to methods for converting gays.

As late as the 1980s, psychiatric hospitals in North America administered electroshock therapy to gays and lesbians to kill the "lust center" in the brain. And today, there are still religious sects and other groups, such as the ex-gay or exodus movement, who actively target gay people to convert them. In these groups, people learn not to accept themselves as they are, and to reject their own desire and love for those of the same sex.

Since the research has so often focused on "curing" gays, there are lots of reasons to be critical of evidence about the "cause" of homosexuality. You'll probably encounter scientists who claim to have found the "gay gene," or psychologists who argue that an overprotective mother is a factor in homosexuality. The evidence always ends up being inconsistent. The basic point is that we don't really know what causes homosexuality. And why is it so important? Why do so many people have a need to explain the origin of homosexuality? Is it because they still have a hard time accepting those who behave differently from the straight norm? The main thing is to make sure that love between any two people is not considered better or worse than love between two others.

How Common Is It?
Have you ever noticed how obsessed some people are with percentages and other numbers? They love using numbers to explain human experience, so they sit around in classrooms and workplaces calculating and preaching about how many gays, Green Party members or cancer victims there are in their community. But sexuality doesn't work the same way as party membership or having a disease. You vote for a party and you succumb to a disease. Sexual boundaries are not as clear and definite. So it's almost impossible to figure out how many people share a certain sexual preference.

One of the most comprehensive and famous studies of sexual habits was done by Alfred Kinsey in the 1940s and 1950s. In the study called *Sexual Behaviour in the Human Male* he presented the following statistics:

- Five percent of all the men studied were purely homosexual and could not imagine having heterosexual sex.
- Ten to thirty percent of all the people he studied preferred homosexual sex for a short or extended period of time.
- Forty percent of all the men studied had had sex with a man that terminated in orgasm.

Kinsey's study caused a shockwave in the American public when it was published in 1948. The idea that almost half of adult American men had had sex with other men was considered unthinkable. Even though later studies have actually shown lower percentages, Kinsey's study is still considered groundbreaking in showing statistically the extent of sexual behavior that isn't "normal."

Kinsey didn't really figure out how many gay people there were, because that is next to impossible. For example, Kinsey's study didn't address love. It only studied sexual habits, and homosexuality is not just about sexual acts. But Kinsey's study did pave the way for more liberated ideas around both straight and gay sex. He pointed out that people can't be divided into two groups, heterosexual and homosexual, like sheep and goats. And nothing is ever black and white. Only humans, Kinsey noted, construct such rigid categories. In real life, it's different — one type blends seamlessly into the other. The sooner we accepted this, Kinsey predicted, the better we'd understand human sexuality.

Max, 19

Actually, I've always been hot for girls. I don't think I've even thought about my own sexuality. It's been pretty much a given. But a while ago, I started to feel almost irritated that my sexuality was so straightforward. I was curious about trying gay sex. Not that I was longing to be with a guy, but because I wanted to try something new. It felt almost abnormal that I had never touched another dick besides my own.

One day while I was watching my friend's basketball game, I ended up sitting next to one of his friends, a guy I'd never met before. Neither one of us was into the game, so we shot the shit instead. We walked home together, and when we got to his place, he asked if I wanted to come up.

We sat on his couch talking (mostly about sex) and drinking. It felt good to suddenly share sexual secrets with someone I'd met just a few hours ago. There was some kind of sexual feeling in the room, and he started kissing me and unzipping my pants. I was kind of nervous and didn't really get hard, so he put a porn movie on. It helped me get that feeling of depravity back, and we continued making out. Really it was the situation that turned me on, not the guy. But it didn't matter. I've never regretted doing it.

Gaybirds and Lezzie-lions

There's one homophobic argument that's sillier than most. You might run into people who hold forth about what's "natural" and "unnatural." They think they know how nature is made up. They might be biologists who think we are preprogrammed for heterosexuality so we can procreate, or they could be Christians who claim that God created man and woman for each other. Sometimes, people use the argument that a woman's sex organs are built to accommodate a penis.

But the truth is, we don't know what's natural. And if God

exists, we can only speculate about why he/she/it planned the world. On the one hand, what we do know is that humans do a whole lot of stuff that doesn't occur in "nature." We have microwaves, cars and iPods. And on the other hand, we know that all this stuff is occurring on the earth, and so it's easy to make the counter-argument that iPods are as "natural" as anything else in the world.

Another "nature" argument, that animals never engage in homosexual sex, is just plain wrong. Today we know that homosexual sex acts are routine among many if not most animal species. There are plenty of gaybirds and lezzie-lions.

"But gay people can't procreate," goes another argument. "Imagine if we all turned gay, the human race would die out." That's just bad logic. Not only is it obvious that homosexuals are a minority and probably always will be, but it's also not true that gay people don't or can't have kids. In fact, it's becoming more common and more accepted for lesbians and gay men to adopt or foster children. The number of lesbians who choose to reproduce by artificial means, that is, using donated sperm, is rising all across the Western world. At the same time, many straight couples choose not to have children.

People talk a lot of garbage. Ask these people to define what they mean by nature. And let them know that they don't get to define what is natural and what isn't. I guarantee that you'll find it easy to beat them at their own game. Promise.

Musty Myths and Pie-in-the-sky Prejudices

"Gay guys are turned on by everyone of the same sex."
This myth that just won't die was obviously created by paranoid homophobes. It's almost ridiculously stupid. Of course gay men are just as picky — or not, as the case may be — as straight people. It should go without saying that loneliness can make you desper-

ate whether you're straight or gay. Most of us lower our standards on occasion, regardless of our sexual orientation. Those who believe in this myth are also likely to chime in with, "Fags are fine, as along as they're not all over me." When someone makes that statement, I always think, "Don't flatter yourself."

"Homosexuality can be cured."
Cure what? Homosexuality is love, sex and tender feelings — not a disease. The idea of "curing" homosexuality has a very sad history: it has often resulted in both mental and physical abuse. Through religious dogma and medical experimentation, societies have terrorized gays in order to "convert" them. Believe me, you do not want to touch this nasty fabrication with a ten-foot pole.

"In a gay relationship, one person plays the woman and the other plays the man."
This is another popular myth that is so outdated it's laughable — and about as true as the one about the stork. In a relationship between two men, they are both — you got it — men.

How Do I Know if I'm Gay?

Around age fourteen, a new question started to pop up more and more often for me. Suddenly I started to wonder whether I was gay or straight. Even though I was smitten with a lot of girls, I brooded my way through sleepless nights and boring science classes. I had nothing against gays, but I'd rather not be one myself. How would I have kids? What would Mom and Dad say? How would they react if I brought a boyfriend home for Sunday night dinner? How would my future nephews and nieces feel about having a gay uncle? Another reason that I was worried I might be gay was that I thought men's bodies were kind of unappealing. I thought I might miss women's breasts and curves. Plus I didn't know how guys had sex with each other. Could I learn? And how would I find other gay men? I read in the paper that guys are usually clear about their sexual orientation at some point during puberty. I waited and waited. I was sure that one day soon, homosexual feelings would wash over me.

In the halls at school, other people seemed to spend a lot of time talking about gay versus straight. Some speculated loudly about how gays behave in bed and what makes "them" tick. The myths were rampant. One friend of mine had a neighbor who was gay and lived with his partner, and my friend was convinced that one person played the woman in the relationship. And everywhere, there were theories about how they "did it."

Looking back, I understand why the interest in homosexuality was so strong during early high school. The obvious reason is that we were all going through the same thing: we were wondering, "Am I gay?" Those who speculated the loudest and had the worst things to say about gays were probably losing the most sleep. Why else were they so obsessed?

I kept wondering about it, but once I started dating some girls more seriously, I realized I actually wasn't gay. Lots of my friends made the same discovery. Others figured out — or already knew — that they were gay or bisexual. Some came out right away in high school; other waited for months or years.

I don't think there's a rule that dictates when you discover your sexuality – not everyone does figure it out during puberty. Several of my gay friends say that they knew much earlier, some not. Some lesbians and gay men remember their first same-sex feelings from nursery school, while others wake up to the reality one day when they're already married, with a house and three kids.

In the best of all worlds, I wouldn't have spent all that time being anxious about my sexual orientation. My preoccupation was founded in the fear of being different or weird — the odd one out. The whole time, I kept hoping that I would end up being turned on by girls so I could be "normal" like everyone else. That's because it's still not easy to be bi or gay in our society. Despite all the progress, you are still expected to fall in love with and be turned on by the opposite sex. Media and other services are still built around the mother-father-child constellation. But things are changing — and the hope is that one day, teens won't need to feel fear or anxiety. It will be completely okay to have sex with girls or guys. We won't necessarily have gay, bi and straight definitions, either. Perhaps we will adopt new expressions for sexuality, hopefully with fewer rules and boundaries attached.

Don't you agree it's a bit strange how fixated people are on labels? Homosexuality and bisexuality are about love and emotions, which are very fluid things.

And you may know people who are transsexual or transgendered. Some people feel that they have been trapped inside the wrong body and are uncomfortable with their sex or gender. For example, a boy may feel that somehow his penis and testicles do not belong to him and he identifies more with having breasts or even a vagina. These men — and women who have the opposite feeling, that they would be more comfortable in a male body — are called transsexual or transgendered. They may make a decision to change their gender, sometimes just by identifying as the other gender, sometimes through surgery and drugs.

And yet, many believe that gays are all a certain way. "Straights are just people, whereas fags are fags," they think. Those people are forgetting that these sexual labels don't necessarily say anything about what or who someone is. They simply describe what gender turns them on.

For most of us, our sexual orientation becomes an obvious fact at a certain point. Usually, you just need to give it some time. But remember, too, that there are straight guys who sometimes have sex with men, and gay men who choose to be celibate. Only you can decide what your sexuality is — it's not determined by what you do. Ultimately, bi, homo and hetero labels are just that — labels. And we'd be living in a very mind-numbing world if there weren't more individual tastes and orientations than there are labels to describe them.

Leonardo, 17

I started thinking about guys some time in grade eight. I was a total macho guy early on in high school, though, and a fag hater on the outside. Inside, I was terrified of being gay. I remember telling my best girlfriend that I thought I was gay, and she hit the roof and was really freaked out. Maybe it's because she was in love with me. I also told two other people, though, and they supported me.

On a school trip when I was fourteen, I got to be really good buddies with another guy. He was amazing and we got along really well. I liked hanging out with him, and he was good-looking and six years older. He was interested in me and I started to think I was in love with him. He was a really good guy and I could relate to him.

I wasn't very self-confident and tried to deny the feelings because I didn't want to be gay. It's probably because I was raised Catholic and because of my mom's views on homosexuality. She doesn't like gays. Mom's brother is gay and her sister is a lesbian, and almost all their friends are gay, too. Mom can't stand them and says they are offensive. She says they are devils. It sounds so eighteenth century when she talks that way. I knew she would be brutally disappointed when I came out. I tried to convince myself to stop thinking about guys. I'd be walking down the street, thinking, "That guy is so hot. Shit." I felt really hesitant and anxious knowing that thoughts like that meant I was gay.

I have some experience kissing guys, both casual kisses, like between friends, and more sexual ones. I've kissed a few guys —

they were all good-looking. A few of them were friends. Some of my female friends are kind of curious about guys kissing.

Six months ago, I came really close to getting a blow job from a guy. An old friend who I don't see that much invited me to a party in another town. I didn't know anyone at the party, so I was sort of being a different person, and was braver than I normally am. Someone introduced me to this guy and right away we were checking each other out and I could feel a connection. We had a few drinks and chatted — we both like jazz. Sitting next to each other on the couch, we started kissing. The girls were mostly egging us on and the other guys didn't seem to care because they were already coupled up with girls. Then we went into a room where some people were making out, and we started making out, too. It felt fine. He felt my dick and I was already hard. He started undoing my zipper and I thought, "Should I do it or not? Isn't it okay to try things and open up a bit?" But when he started to grab my dick, I couldn't do it, it didn't feel right. I told him it wasn't working. He was kind of pissed off. He was really hot, though, he could've been a model.

I recently met a girl who I'm in love with, so I've stopped thinking about guys as much. I don't think I want to be with a guy in the future. I know I would feel guilty in front of my mom. I'm sure I can get by without it. But definitely, if you fall in love, you fall in love, and that's that — you can't stop love. If I start having feelings for a guy, I won't stop them. I wouldn't hide it if I really fell in love.

Coming Out

You're already aware that guys turn you on. There's no question that you're gay. You're clear about your sexual orientation. But maybe you haven't told anyone yet. Maybe you find it tedious when your guy friends constantly talk about girls. Everywhere there are people asking you if you've found a girlfriend. Your family, friends and siblings are endlessly curious. And they all assume that you're into girls. Either you play along, or you avoid the subject with your questioning aunts and with your buddies who constantly razz you about the girl they're convinced you had something going on with at camp last summer.

Maybe you're thinking about telling people about your sexuality. You weigh the alternatives: are you better off hiding it for a while longer, or should you just bite the bullet? But how is the larger world going to react? What will your mom, your friends and your siblings have to say? Your dad and your friends may have made a few gay jokes. So will they turn their back, get angry, be stunned into silence, or support you in your sexuality?

Before coming out about your homo- or bisexuality, I think it's a good idea to be as sure as you can be of your preferences. And as difficult as it might be, try to work on accepting yourself: the reality is that it's more difficult for others to accept you if you don't accept yourself. Preparing yourself for the questions others might ask you is also a good idea.

The history of coming out as gay and telling your community is something that all openly gay people share. It's a history that's riddled with fear, anxiety and grief, but it's also about the fantastic feeling of relief and liberation that comes with not having anything to hide anymore. Your most important resource in preparing to come out is other out gay people: seek them and ask for their support and advice.

You probably have lots of questions to ask and probably carry around lots of thoughts you need to bounce off other gay people. Hopefully you know a gay person you can talk to. Maybe someone in your school is already out. But only turn to them if they seem trustworthy. You will also be able to find community resources. If you live in a big city, find out where the gay area is and go there to look for the local community center. If you live in a smaller community, the Internet will help you connect with a virtual community of support. You can phone local or national gay and bisexual help lines from anywhere in the US and Canada. These services are free and anonymous, and many are especially for youth. Use these resources to connect with other gay people in your area.

When you feel ready, you just have to pick a time to speak up. The first person you tell should be someone you feel close to and who you think will handle the news well, such as a best friend or a sibling. Or if you can't bring yourself to talk to the person face to face, write them a letter instead. Once you've told one person, the next step will feel easier.

Often, the reactions are less dramatic than you might have imagined. After all, in the Western world, homosexuality is both widespread and legally accepted. But some people are simply intolerant. Chances are that at least one of the people who you thought would be fine with your news will react with shock or anger. That reaction should make you think: if someone is angry with me when I have just taken the step of trying to be honest with them, is that person a good friend? The answer is no. If this person can't respect your sexuality, their friendship isn't worth very much. Friendship can't be built on narrow-mindedness and insularity.

Most parents aren't overjoyed when their kids come out as gay or bi. Expecting champagne and balloons is unrealistic. Even if parents are tolerant, they are usually worried. That said, very few parents stop loving their kids because they're gay. When you tell your parents, they might be so surprised at first that they can't think of what to say. Give them some time to process the information and formulate the questions they need answers to. In the same way that it took you a while to figure out and accept your sexuality, it will take your parents some time, too. They might need just five minutes, or, more commonly, days, weeks – or even a month.

Coming out isn't a one-time occurrence. Telling your parents and some close friends is probably just the beginning: you will have to explain things to them over again, and there will always be more people to come out to. But if you've come out once, you'll be less afraid of doing it again. Once you feel acceptance from even one person who is close to you, you will have support to fall back on. As an openly gay person, there are always more people to come out to: new friends, your church community, your co-workers. The list might seem endless. But although coming out never really ends, it is also a gradual process. Coming out to those who are two steps removed from your private life, such as your doctor, your guidance counselor, your extended family and your friend's parents, will happen in time.

When people you encounter ask if you have a girlfriend, you can choose how you want to answer. When and if you tell others that you're interested in guys is completely up to you. Be prepared to go on answering questions — some of them irritating or just downright stupid — from everyone you have already come out to, as well. No matter what happens, it's always better to have taken some steps toward coming out. Living in the closet can be isolating and easily leads to a wide range of negative feelings.

Society is gradually getting easier for gay men and lesbians. Fewer and fewer people reject homosexuality, and typical questions around dating and relationships have started to change; more and more people will ask if you have met "someone" as opposed to a girl. And at some point in the future, people you meet will stop assuming that you and everyone else are straight.

Being openly gay was not an option until quite recently. Closeted lesbians and gays battled with heavy burdens of shame and guilt. Many were forced to repress or hide their desire, even from themselves. Many gay men ended up in unhappy marriages with women they didn't desire. Thankfully, if you are young and gay today, you do have options. If you are thinking of coming out or have made any first tentative steps, remind yourself that there is a whole amazing world out there waiting for you. As a young gay person, you can look forward to finding wonderful new friends, sexual experiences and love. You will realize that you are absolutely not alone as a gay person in the world today.

Simon, 23

Looking back now, I can tell that I've probably been gay my whole life. Around age twelve or thirteen, I started to realize that I was attracted to guys, but I thought it was a phase. At scout's camp, I met a girl from another city who was crazy good-looking. We almost kissed and I wanted to get together with her so badly, to prove to myself that it could work with a girl and that I was straight.

I tried having relationships with girls until my second year of high school, but then I got it that I was a fag. But I just couldn't say it. I didn't think about the future. There were no other gay men, at least none that I knew of. I had no one to talk to. It felt like there was no way I could be gay in my school. Homosexuality didn't even exist in school, it seemed. It's not like I was thinking, "What would happen if I told someone?" I just didn't believe that I could lead a gay life. That would mean finding a boyfriend — meeting guys, dating, making out or having sex with them — but there were no guys. What guys would that be? I didn't see any opportunities. Since I couldn't be a practicing gay guy anyway, I thought I might as well not tell anyone.

But when I got into my second year of high school, I told my best friend. Then I came out to our closest circle of friends. We had talked about things like that, so I knew that they would be open. In junior high and early high school, I had hung out with the cool crowd, where the guys were seriously macho. But in grade ten, I was drawn to friends who I generally had more in common with and who were more into the arts, like theater. And it was lucky for me that I happened to be gay and interested in culture, because I found that artsy people are often more open and progressive. If I had been interested in car racing, I might not have come out, actually.

The worst was coming out to my family. Friends come and go, but you're stuck with your family. When you face them, everything feels way more complicated.

I had planned it for a long time, and I tried to drop hints by talking about related things. I started mentioning gay rights in political discussions at dinner, and one day I told my parents I had become friends with a gay guy and was going with him to a gay club. Later that night my dad asked half-jokingly if I was gay. I was kind of freaked out by that, because I had been planning to sit them down and talk to them for real. My mom totally broke down because she thought Dad was being a klutz, so her first reaction was to turn to my dad and start screaming at him, "What the hell are you saying to our son??" I had never heard my parents use language like that with each other, so I thought I was causing a rift in their marriage.

But really, they were just worried about me. They thought things would be difficult for me and they were afraid that people would give me a hard time. And I guess in some ways that's true, because it is tougher to be gay than straight. You are definitely part of a small minority. You have to explain your sexuality and come out to new people all the time. You don't always want to "be" your sexuality to everyone you meet.

That's why there's gay culture. Gay culture exists because gay people have been forced to identify with their sexuality because they have been discriminated against.

That's why gay people have been able to find support through building up a community of common interests. But really, there aren't that many commonalities between gay people. What do we have in common? Basically, the fact that we have sex with people of the same gender. That's it. Period. There is no gay gene that makes us all like Barbra Streisand. It's a total pain when people mix all those things together. They make a mess of reality. People who don't know any gay men think that homosexuality is connected to your taste in music, or that talking with a feminine voice means that you're gay, which is so not true. The worst thing is that I sometimes fall for the stereotypes, too. They're hard to get away from.

How Do Gay Guys Have Sex?

There's one obvious advantage to being gay. Sex. As a homosexual man, you don't have to bother with figuring out how to unhook a bra or find the clitoris. You never have to worry about accidental pregnancy, either. You know what pleasures you, so it's probably not that hard to figure out what gets your guy off. Your bodies are usually built just about the same.

Most people think that gay guys have anal sex constantly. That there's nothing they love more. In reality, anal sex isn't as common among gays as you might think. The hetero assumption that gay men are anal sex fanatics is based on the heterosexual view of sex. In short, for a lot of straight people, sex is defined by one thing: penetration. But in actual fact, that's pretty simple-minded, considering the amazing range of sexual activities that our bodies offer us. There are so many things you can do. Jerking each other off and sucking each other off are just two of the possibilities. If you've ever masturbated, you know how to jerk a guy off. Do what you would do to your own penis, but be sensitive to his reactions. He might like it harder or faster, softer or slower. A good way to make sure the other person is enjoying himself is as simple as asking, "Does that feel good?" or using little questions like, "Harder?" or "Faster?"

Sucking someone off is another way to say oral sex, that is, sex with your mouth. Oral sex between men entails sucking on the other guy's penis. You suck carefully, not hard, like on a candy. The principle is the same as when you jerk someone or yourself off, but the difference is, you do it with your mouth. Make sure to open your mouth wide, and keep your teeth away from the penis – otherwise, it can be very painful. Improvise, play with your tongue, and do whatever else you think feels good. Too far in, and the penis can make you gag. The best rule is to stick with your own comfort level.

Anal sex involves stimulation in and around the rectum. You can use your fingers, your penis or other objects. Since the rectum is sensitive and tight, caution is required when having anal sex. (Read more about anal sex in Chapter 13.)

Chapter 7
Masturbation

The summer between grades three and four, I went to sailing camp. We sailed, had campfires and made up rude songs about each other in our cabins at night. I was the youngest person at camp and got to learn a lot more than just sailing and camp songs. One day my friend Jens told me about pulling and stroking my penis until something white came out. It felt good when I tried it, but the white stuff never came. For that reason it felt a bit like a failed chemistry experiment, but I was happy to have learned something that felt so good. I turned into a diligent masturbator, and a couple of years later, the white stuff arrived, too — sperm. The experiment was complete.

Historically in the West, masturbation has been considered bad, dirty and even harmful. As early as 300 BC, Aristophanes, who was a Greek playwright, said that masturbation as an activity was ill-suited to men. He said it was more fitting for women, children, slaves and weak old men. But the really intensive campaign against masturbation didn't start until the 1700s. In 1710, *Onania* was published, most likely authored by a theologian called Balthasar Bekker. Earlier, masturbation had meant interrupted intercourse, but now it came to mean sexual self-pleasuring. *Onania* depicted masturbators as potential victims of spinal decay, sterility, gonorrhea, impotence, epilepsy and stunted growth.

Doctors and teachers joined theologians like Bekker in the fight against masturbation, so the theory that masturbation caused damage had both religious and scientific foundations. *Onania* was just the beginning of a flood of books and so-called studies that opposed masturbation.

During the 1900s, the propaganda against masturbation slowly died out. Doctors realized that it was harmless, but many still considered it sinful.

Today, the vast majority of people consider masturbation completely safe, but there are still a few groups that believe otherwise. A few fundamentalist faiths teach that masturbation is sinful and egotistical. I have thought about it through and through, but I can't make heads or tails of their point of view. Wouldn't brushing your teeth and clipping your nails be considered just as selfish then? Those are also things we do in private, for their own sake.

In general, I believe that it's more harmful to feel guilty about jerking off than to jerk off with a carefree attitude. What's the point of carrying around all that guilt over something that is a perfectly natural, safe and pleasurable behavior?

The Bible doesn't actually say anything about masturbation being bad or dangerous, at least in its modern meaning. The Biblical character who embodied early Christian views on masturbation was Onan, who spilled his seed. Be aware, though, that Onan didn't spill his seed by jerking off, as many believe, but through interrupted intercourse, which was apparently highly unpopular with God (at least according to the authors of the Bible).

Masturbation entails sexual self-pleasuring, that is, touching yourself so that you feel pleasure. The most common way for circumcised men to masturbate is to stroke the shaft up and down with their fingers or hands until orgasm. Uncircumcised men typically pull the foreskin back and forth to reach orgasm.

Jerking off is fantastic because you can do it any time you

want. A quick session in the bathroom or a long evening in your bedroom with dimmed lights and good music on. A little jerk-off session before dropping off to sleep can be a great way to relax. It feels wonderful, it's free — and you don't have to ask anyone for permission.

Besides the penis, you can also touch yourself anywhere else it feels good while masturbating. Some people like touching their scrotum, their nipples, their butt cheeks or their anus. When it comes to masturbation, nothing is wrong. You get to jerk off as much or as little as you want. Jerking off can't harm you, no matter how much you do it. If you are going through a very intense period of masturbation, you may get little blisters or cuts. They aren't dangerous and will heal on their own after a few days. If it hurts to jerk off, it's a good idea to wait until the pain is gone before you try again.

Some people use stimulatory aids like movies, magazines or novels when they jerk off. Others make the fantasies up in their head. In your fantasies, you get to go anywhere you want. So you don't have to feel ashamed if some odd things pop up in your fantasies. It's not weird if your teacher, aunt or best friend come up. Fantasies are sort of like dreams. They help you work out things that happen to you in life. Fantasizing about someone does not necessarily mean that you want her or him in real life. That's why it's also not unusual to fantasize about someone other than your steady partner, if you have one. You see the partner all the time anyway. Fantasy scenarios are often about what's unattainable or hard to come by. So fantasizing is a great way to explore reality without any consequences.

You also don't have to stop jerking off when you commit to a relationship or a specific sexual partner. Commitment and masturbation are not mutually exclusive. Masturbation is your own thing, and you should do it whenever you feel like it.

Guys often talk unabashedly about their masturbation,

whereas girls are sometimes quieter about what happens sexually when they're alone. Be advised that this doesn't mean that girls jerk off less than guys. Sometimes they don't talk about masturbating because women's sexuality is still more taboo than male sexuality. Even now, girls are likely to learn at an early age that their sexuality — especially any enjoyment they may have on their own time – should be concealed or even repressed.

People of all ages have a hard time accepting that women and girls experience their own, independent sexual desire and pleasure, even though it's now blatantly clear that their sexual needs are just as strong and present as men's. One outdated view of women's sexuality was that women didn't feel pleasure during sex but more or less put up with it in order to please their spouse and get pregnant. The reasons for this theory are pretty complicated, and I can't even start to explain them in this book. But I'm hoping you agree that this attitude is so obviously ridiculous that it's amazing that anyone could have truly believed it.

How Do Girls Jerk Off?

What actually happens in girls' bedrooms, toilets and showers? Is it rubbing, massaging, stroking or penetrating? Hard, soft or both? Sorry, I have no definite answers here. Not to sound like a cliché, but there are just as many female masturbation techniques as there are women. Every girl has her own technique. In general, the most common way for a girl to masturbate is to rub on and around the clitoral area with her fingers. Orgasm, which is usually, but not always, the goal of masturbation, can be attained in several ways: clitoral or vaginal stimulation, as well as any variation or combination of both. The majority of women and girls reach orgasm through clitoral stimulation rather than vaginal stimulation alone. Some girls like to rub their clit hard, whereas others like it as soft as a flutter. Some girls rub right on the clitoris itself, whereas others are more sensitive and rub the hood, or above or below the clit. The method can also vary from day to day — just like it might for you or other guys. Some days you might stroke hard, and other days a soft touch feels best.

Vaginal masturbation means masturbation with penetration, which means inserting something into the vagina. Penetration can stimulate the G-spot, which is located higher up along the frontal vaginal wall and is actually more like an area than a spot. Penetration can also stimulate the clitoris indirectly by pulling and rubbing the clitoral hood.

Girls sometimes use dildos to masturbate, for penetration and for clitoral stimulation. Reaching the G-spot can be challenging and a dildo can help with that, too. Instead of buying expensive masturbation aids, many girls use what they can find in the house, like candles, cucumbers, carrots or deodorant bottles, or whatever feels good and has the right size and shape. Some girls insert fingers or a dildo into the vagina while they are rubbing the clitoris, but just as many don't insert anything at all. Another way girls jerk off is by rubbing or pressing against something, with or without underwear on. Still other girls jerk off in the shower using a showerhead.

The main masturbation principle for girls is the same as it is for guys: they touch themselves whenever, wherever and whichever way feels good.

Chapter 8
Porn

Cum shots, spread-eagled women, silicone implants, bad plots, mustaches, lingerie and tube socks. Simply put, ready-made fantasies for when you can't find the energy to fantasize.

It's time to talk porn, a subject that seems to engage almost everyone. Some people are against porn: they're offended by the scripted sex acts on display. Others say they're against porn... and feel guilty that they can't help secretly consuming it. And still other people think that porn is an unbeatable tool for masturbating. A select few even try to turn their porn use into an acceptable hobby by collecting specific kinds of porn, like, say, 1960s porn or French porn. And still others use porn for educational purposes.

According to the dictionary, the word pornography means "the explicit description or exhibition of sexual activity in literature, films, etc. intended to stimulate erotic rather than aesthetic or emotional feelings," and stems from the Greek *pornographos*, meaning "writing about prostitutes." People have always made pictures of humans having sex, and yet, pornography has always been a more or less controversial topic. And so it is to this day.

During the 1960s, the North American market in pornography exploded because of the sexual liberation movements. Led by such high-profile advocates as John Lennon and Yoko Ono, a growing portion of North Americans started to adopt more liberal attitudes toward sex. As more people got better access to birth control, the idea of sex for pleasure became more accepted. This led many to argue for an end to censorship of sexual imagery, in order to open the door for talented artists, writers and filmmakers to make porn. The idea was that if porn were brought up from its underground status, its quality would improve. What happened instead? Well, all of these changes encouraged a huge growth in pornography as a highly profitable industry. Large numbers of peep shows opened, where men masturbated while watching porn. With the arrival of the video player, porn saw another huge upswing — suddenly, porn movies could be consumed in private. More recently, the Internet and digital television have given porn even more substantial boosts. Today, the porn industry is one of the world's largest industries. All this porn was and is made mostly by and for men and, in the early 1970s, women's movements started protesting against the porn industry as being sexist and degrading toward women.

The climate for porn was different in Canada than in the US. In general, Canadian sexual liberation movements were less powerful than those in the US, and the courts were less accommodating: many Canadian citizens believed pornography could be harmful both to those making porn and to those consuming it. In the 1980s, these citizens began pressuring lawmakers to outlaw violent and degrading pornography. In the 1985 case *R. v. Towne Cinema*, the Supreme Court of Canada adopted the view that pornography degrades and dehumanizes women, and as a result, pornography is less extensively available in Canada than it is in the United States. However, the restrictions on pornography in Canada and the US have not gone unchallenged, and today, many Canadians and Americans believe that porn is a normal and acceptable part of their sex lives.

What do you think about porn?

Eric, 16
I know that what you use porn for is to get turned on. You don't need it when you have a girlfriend... well, maybe sometimes. I watch porn now and then. Really, I feel sorry for the girls in the movies, and the weirdest thing is that I don't care, I just watch it anyway.

Leo, 17
I have nothing against porn. Pornos are fun for the first fifteen minutes, and then it's the same thing over and over again. Cheap thrills!

John, 19
When I was younger it felt cool to watch porn but now I've gotten sick of it. It feels so boring and fake! Just in, out and squirt. I can't say I get much out of porn.

My First Porn Mag
Middle school. My friend and I have decided we're going to buy a porn mag. For some reason, I'm chosen to do the deed. My friend stands guard on the slushy sidewalk outside the convenience store. I almost pee my pants from the tension, shame and anxiety. The line-up is long and I do everything I can to hide what I'm buying. I only have small change to pay with and the line grows behind me. My cheeks burn. But the feeling when I pull the magazine out of my backpack later is awesome. I wonder what the tingling and shivering is all about. The pictures make me almost dizzy.

As I looked for the first time at these naked women who, in spreading their legs and arching their backs, expressed a kind of fierce hunger, very intense feelings awakened in me. My newly purchased magazine became a ticket to my own private sexuality. And to other people's sexuality. It felt as far away from my parents' wholesome affection for each other as I could ever get. And it awakened feelings of fear, fascination and that tingling I didn't have a name for yet. It was a whole new perspective on the proper, orderly adult world.

I was, quite simply, aroused — and that's probably the way it is for most porn consumers. Basically, you get turned on when you see naked people having sex. Lots of sex, totally free from love and responsibility. In porn, sex is for everyone. The men often (but not always) have potbellies and pasty skin, but they still get to have sex with large-breasted, slim blondes. And the girls want to go again and again. In porn, no one says they're not in the mood, or that they feel hurt or that they're pregnant. In this way, porn is a kind of erotic dreamscape where ugly, rejected men are vindicated. Sometimes, porn is violent and degrading. It's as if by watching other women be manhandled, the porn consumer is exacting revenge on all the women who ever dissed him.

Porn as Sex Instructor

When I was in grade seven, it hit me that at some point I should prepare myself for my first sexual escapade. I realized I needed some sexual instruction. Dusty biology books didn't have the answers I needed, so I decided I should start watching pornos. I had seen some snippets of movies before, but this time I was going to be much more analytical and perceptive. I was going to study how this whole sex thing worked. Which hole was where, how you thrust, what rhythm you should use, and so on. Thankfully, my studies never took off. I couldn't work up the courage to rent any porn movies, and my parents probably would have noticed if I sat up watching the pay TV channels late at night. Time passed, and one day, my sexual debut arrived without the preparation I had intended. Now, in retrospect, I'm very happy about that.

In fact, watching porn for educational purposes is an exceptionally foolish way to prepare for your first sexual experience. Sex in the pornographic world is one thing and sex in the real world is something completely different. And besides, you can't really learn how to have sex. You can study what various body parts and erogenous zones are called and where they're located, but you can never practice a sexual experience ahead of time (unless you do it with your partner). Because when you have sex with another person, you create the conditions of your encounter together. If you've already decided in advance what you're going to do with your partner, there's no interaction. You might as well just jerk off. The cool thing about sex is getting turned on together. That doesn't happen if there's a porn movie director in your bed. When one person decides on the positions and calls the shots, what you get is a one-sided experience, not a mutual zone where you turn each other on.

If you think porn tells the truth about sex, then you think girls get off on being told what to do in bed. You believe that the standard penis size is twenty-three centimeters (nine inches) and that it's normal to come on a girl's face. You think all girls have huge round boobs that stand straight up when they're lying on their backs. You think girls love to give blow jobs and that anal sex is uncomplicated or a given. You think it's okay to put your penis straight into the vagina from the anus without washing it first. Basically, if you think porn is even close to reality, you have a lot of things completely backwards. The fact that porn is different from the bedroom is what makes it so exciting. Much of what you see in porn is there because it looks good on film. That's why the guys come on the girls' chests and faces: the sperm has to be visible. Porn consumers want to see things that are cruder and rougher than what they do with their own partner. Sure, there are girls in the real world who like to give head, have breast implants and like anal sex. But in the world of porn, those things are the rule rather than the exception.

Porn also portrays a crappy, outdated view of women and men. It's the bully caveman making all the decisions for the submissive cavewoman. He groans and pumps while she squeals. Suddenly, he pulls out and sprays all over her. In pornos, women basically never reach orgasm. The woman turns into a tool for the man's pleasure. In reality, men are no longer bullies and women are not doormats that they step all over. When you look at it this way, porn is insulting to both men and women.

People who watch porn must feel stressed and pressured if they believe that this is how they should perform sexually. And just as many people must be surprised or disappointed when they figure out that sex isn't what they've been watching on their X-rated videos. I feel sorry for both kinds of people, because they don't get this basic fact: sex is about making decisions along with your partner about trying things that are fun and exciting. It's not what you've seen online or in your tattered *Hustler* magazine. It's okay to do whatever you want in bed, as long as both of you help decide what to do. Porn shouldn't decide for you, and neither should anyone else, for that matter.

Using porn as a how-to guide for sex is about as smart and useful as using kung fu movies to get ready for your trip to Asia, or using *Law and Order* to study for a law degree.

Also, be aware that it's obvious to girls if they're having sex with a guy who has watched porn to prepare his performance. At least that's what Tanya, Sasha and Debbie said. (All three were just graduating from high school when I interviewed them.) They weren't against porn, but they thought that porn has a strange influence on guys and that there's a lot of bad stuff in it.

Are men affected by porn movies?
Tanya: Yes, I think they are. If you aren't in touch with your own individual sexuality, you'll be influenced by all the images that you see in porn. It's scary what a narrow picture porn gives of sex. It's

most harmful for people who watch it to educate themselves. Most guys I know have had an intense experience with porn at some point and, of course, that affects you.

Can you tell when you're having sex with a guy who has watched a lot of porn?
Sasha: Definitely! One guy I had sex with pulled my hair and kept moving me around in different positions even though he was a virgin. It was very clear where he had learned that stuff. Guys who have watched lots of porn think sex follows a specific pattern, as if there's a manual or something.
Tanya: People who use porn as an instruction manual lose their ability to use their senses. They forget the girl's pleasure and try to pack in as many extreme scenarios as they can during sex. It turns into an act instead of bodies turning each other on. Sex like that is about asserting control and making the grade. Some guys even use terms from porn to evaluate the sex they've had.

Can you see any good sides to porn?
Tanya: Sure, if you already feel good about your sexuality and understand how narrow porn is, you can take what you want from it instead of being manipulated.
Debbie: But in a good sexual relationship, you shouldn't need porn to try new, exciting things. After all, human beings are animals and have a natural tendency to explore different ways to get pleasure.

What else don't you like about it then?
Tanya: It's pretty bad that porn sets out such limited roles and unrealistic demands on youth who are at the beginning of their sex lives. Girls never say no and guys are always hard. Otherwise, something's wrong. And men are almost always dominant in porn. If the woman is ever on top, it's always the man who's decided.

Debbie: It's gross with all those fake tans and heavy make-up under such harsh, sterile lighting. And I hate that the norm for being sexy is shaving and having a boob job.

Tanya: It's sad, too, that porn has violated lesbian sex. You can tell how some guys glorify something that they actually have no part in. Some men seem to believe that lesbian sex is a threesome. I've been to parties where guys totally out of the blue encourage straight girls to get it on.

Do you watch porn?

Tanya: Sure, I've watched snippets of porn, but never an entire movie. What turns me on is that it's forbidden, but then after a few minutes I realize I'm watching real people and then I just can't discount the disgusting part of it.

Sasha: I used to watch porn. I wanted to know why people kept telling me it was so awful. Most high school-aged girls I know have watched at least a few pornos. But I personally find it hard to get turned on when I think about the film team shouting instructions and sticking cameras so close to the actors.

Have you been affected by porn?

Tanya: Yeah, I think I've been a bit damaged by it. Some porn scenes have gotten stuck in my head. If a guy I'm with wants to do anything that reminds me of those scenes, I say stop. I can't do it.

What is typical for a girl who's influenced by porn?

Debbie: I think she feels that there are a lot of demands. She has to get turned on immediately and be totally willing. And she has to shave and have perfect make-up on.

Chapter 9
Contraception

You've most likely heard about contraception in school – how to prevent pregnancy. Many guys think that contraception is up to girls. After all, they're the ones who get pregnant. But since guys are just as involved in having sex as girls, they should be just as concerned about pregnancy as the girls are. Who wants to deal with all the responsibilities of fathering a child before they're ready?

There are many different types of contraception, and they're a bit complicated to sort out. Luckily, you only need to know about one simple trick, so you don't have to think about them very much. If you follow this, you'll be fine. Use a condom. Then you don't need to worry — about pregnancy or about sexually transmitted infections (for more on STIs, see Chapter 10). It's such a simple rule to follow that you don't even have to think about it.

Condoms

The condom is the easiest, most perfect security blanket: that's why people have been using condom-type contraception for millennia. Two thousand years ago, the Chinese used oiled rice paper as protection. Since then, people all over the world have invented variations of the condom. Casanova, the seventeenth-century king of seduction, was a religious condom-wearer. At that time, condoms were made of linen or animal intestines. Not very appealing maybe, but Casanova sure loved his condoms; he had a series of endearments for them, including "the English riding coat," "the security kit" and "the English clothes that lend the spirit rest."

Not everyone was as pumped about condoms as Casanova. Condoms were long kept under wraps. In the Western world, laws against birth control, including condoms, weren't overturned until the 1940s, and it was prohibited to buy and sell condoms openly until the 1960s. We are incredibly lucky that condoms are so accessible today, often totally free of charge from your doctor or local medical center. And of course, there are condoms for sale at every little corner store.

There are still guys who feel that condoms are a pain in the neck. Some think a condom takes away some of the sensation, others worry what their partner thinks, and others just feel awkward and clumsy when they have to deal with the condom thing in the midst of all those great horny feelings.

To the guy who thinks it takes away some of the sensation

Today's condoms are so thin they don't affect the sensation very much at all. On the one hand, it's true that it's not exactly the same with a condom as without. On the other hand, condoms actually help guys who suffer from premature ejaculation. If you're someone who thinks that condoms take away some of your pleasure, check your priorities and ask yourself some questions. Is the risk of pregnancy and STIs less important than that little bit of extra enjoyment that condom-free sex brings? Is it worth risking your own health and life or someone else's for a small amount of pleasure? With those questions circling in your head, something is out of whack if you still don't want to use a condom.

To the guy who worries what his partner thinks

Often people have sex without a condom even though they both actually want to be protected. Both partners want to talk about using a condom, but they feel that it's lame to bring it up. So they have a good time, but later, the anxiety starts.

I've sometimes heard guys talk about girls who don't want to use a condom, while they themselves want to. Just as often, I hear girls say exactly the same thing. I suspect that in fact, true resistance to condoms isn't very prevalent. Most people want to protect themselves and they know that condoms are the most reliable way to be safe. That's why you should just bite the bullet and bring it up. And chances are, no one will say no to the idea.

To the guy who feels awkward and clumsy

Everything is at the peak of amazing horniness. Your body is quivering. Intercourse is getting closer, and so is the condom moment. Then it can feel strange and clumsy to start prying open a condom package and playing around to get it on. But your clumsiness can be fixed easily enough: as the saying goes, practice makes perfect.

A great opportunity is when you're masturbating. Since you can get free condoms all over the place, it's not expensive. The method is as follows: unravel the condom slightly to see which direction you should roll it on. Then, pinch the pointy end and roll the rest over the head and down the penis shaft, all the way to the bottom. The pointy end is the sperm sac, and you need to pinch it to make sure it doesn't fill with air.

With a few practice sessions under your belt, you'll be an expert in no time. Then there are other things to consider. If you think your make-out session will lead to intercourse, it can be good to have condoms close at hand. Even better, put them within arm's reach. Traipsing around naked with a big boner while you search for your condoms just doesn't look or feel sexy.

When you pull your penis out after intercourse is over, it's really important to hold the bottom of the condom so it doesn't slide off. Otherwise, the sperm can escape their sac, which is meant to hold them in place.

When a Condom Breaks

When you grab milk out of the fridge, you check the best-before date. The same goes for condoms, because they also last for only a limited time. And if you store a condom in your wallet, you should change it even more often than the best-before date tells you to. The condom gets worn faster when it's mixed in with all those cards, coins and (if you're lucky) bills. If you use an old condom, it can break easily, even when you only have sex for a short time.

Condoms can also break if you have sex for a very long time, or if your partner isn't very wet. Some condoms are lubricated, which might help in those cases. You can use a water-based lubricant with condoms, but don't use oil-based products like petroleum jelly, baby oil or hand cream with latex condoms because they break down the latex. If you come inside the girl and she isn't protected in any other way, there is a risk that she will get pregnant.

Emergency Contraception

The risk of pregnancy can be offset by emergency contraception, or what is also called the morning-after pill. Depending on the type, the morning-after pill can be taken up to 72 hours after unprotected intercourse. The morning-after pill shouldn't be taken lightly, because common side effects include severe nausea. Also, it can be used only once during each menstrual cycle. That's why using emergency contraception instead of regular contraception is not an option.

When your partner has to take the morning-after pill, I think it's important to be there for her. Be supportive and offer to go with her to the drugstore or the clinic. You both had sex, so you should both take responsibility for it.

Interrupted Intercourse

Interrupted intercourse, or pulling out, is when you pull your penis out of the vagina before coming. Throughout history, people have tried to avoid pregnancy using this method. The thing is, it doesn't work very well.

The major problems with this method are as follows: first, it's impossible to know exactly when you should pull out since you have pre-cum, which contains sperm and comes out without warning. Second, it's often very challenging to pull out when your pleasure is at its peak, even if you have the best intentions. This method is certainly better than nothing – but you can't be sure it will always work.

Rhythm Method

Another really unreliable method for avoiding pregnancy is to stick to "safe periods." This means having sex during the few days of your partner's menstrual cycle when the risk of fertilization is the lowest. Specifically, that would mean the few days after her period. The problem is that lots of girls and women have irregular periods, so it's hard to know when ovulation occurs. In other words, the "safe periods" aren't very safe at all.

The Pill

The pill protects against pregnancy by preventing ovulation and making the mucous membrane in the fallopian tubes too thick for the sperm to get through. The pill contains a combination of the female hormones estrogen and progesterone. The pill can also be beneficial for some girls who experience severe menstrual pain, since it regulates the cycle and can reduce or eliminate menstrual symptoms. But like most medications, the pill can have some pretty bad side effects for some girls, including mood swings, weight gain and reduced libido.

Peter, 17

I know a lot more about the pill than my current girlfriend. If we agree that she should be on the pill, I have to know how it works, too. When my last girlfriend told me she was on the pill, we talked a lot about it, and she was psyched that I knew so much about it. If the girl is going to take it, I should know just as much as she does. Also, for me it's a given that the guy should pay for half of the medication.

Chapter 10
Sexually Transmitted Infections

Sexually transmitted infections (STIs) have been around since the earliest recorded human history. Gonorrhea was a topic of discussion in old Egyptian papyrus texts. Although it is easy to cure gonorrhea today, there was a time when people feared this and other diseases, coloring their perception of sex and the people who got these "sinful" diseases. Being afflicted with an STI was a great source of shame. Even today, there are still people who feel that sexually transmitted infections are a punishment from God. In this chapter, I talk about the most common STIs, as well as a particularly dangerous one, HIV. When I had sex ed, it seemed like the teachers and the textbooks wanted us to come away scared. The main message I got was, "Be afraid, be very, very afraid…of sex." Part of me thought, why take the seemingly huge risk of having sex?

This message doesn't reflect reality, though. Remember, with a condom you can protect yourself effectively against almost all STIs. If you use condoms properly and consistently, there's no reason to go around feeling scared.

But if you don't use condoms and have not been tested for all the usual suspects, you need to start using them and get tested (if either of you have had sexual relations before, including oral and anal sex). Many STIs, including HIV, have no symptoms. If you do have symptoms, get yourself to a doctor right away. STIs happen to lots of people. Bacterial infections like chlamydia, gonorrhea and syphilis can be cured with antibiotics. There is also treatment for STIs like herpes, genital warts and HIV/AIDS, which are caused by viruses. This is not something you want to procrastinate about — you could save yourself and your partner(s) a lot of pointless pain and risk.

Chlamydia

When my sister went off to university in another city, she moved into residence. Her residence housed loads of students who mostly kept busy eating ramen noodles and spending endless hours at the library. But all the girls in the residence were fascinated with an art student — let's call him D — who lived in a studio on the top floor of the residence, particularly because he was a painter and a gourmet cook. It slowly became clear that portraits and cooking weren't his only pastimes.

Within a few weeks, several girls from the residence bumped into each other at the campus medical clinic. Some of them start-

Chlamydia Fact Sheet

Symptoms: The symptoms, if there are any, usually appear two to six weeks or longer after infection. You may have a burning sensation when you pee, or in some cases, discharge from the penis or anus. Only about half the men who get chlamydia show symptoms – but you can still infect others, even without symptoms.

Testing: Urine test. This means you pee in a cup. No swabs from the opening at the tip of the penis are necessary unless you have discharge.

Treatment: Antibiotics.

Related Diseases: Untreated chlamydia can lead to infertility in girls, and sometimes in guys as well. If you already have chlamydia, it is easier to get HIV from an infected partner.

ed to exchange stories, and realized that all the girls who had had sex with D had been infected with chlamydia — and it quickly became apparent that this included most girls living in that particular residence.

Herpes

Daniel, 19

It was my first real relationship and we were totally in love and hot for each other. It was the Christmas holidays, and we'd been having a lot of sex. A few days later, we were supposed to borrow my family's cottage outside the city and have it all to ourselves. The only problem was that I had been noticing some itching and burning down there, and so had she.

We had an awesome few days. We made out, made fires and walked across the lake on the ice. It was cold and clear, and the ice was perfectly smooth, like it is when the lake freezes over fast.

We were used to having a lot of sex, especially when we were

Herpes Fact Sheet

Symptoms: Small blisters on the genitals that burn, sting or itch. These are often misdiagnosed or underdiagnosed because they don't look like cold sores. These blisters can take ten to fourteen days to heal. Most of the time, a person gets the virus from someone who has no symptoms.

Testing: If there are blisters, a sample can be taken and sent to the lab for testing. This is useful, because there are a number of STIs with similar symptoms. There is also a lab test to tell whether a person has HSV-1 or HSV-2 on the genitals.

Treatment: Herpes can be treated either during an outbreak or on a regular basis to keep you from infecting others. Herpes stays in your body and can't be cured, but some people find that their outbreaks decrease in strength over time.

alone. But this time, we couldn't. It would have hurt too much. So even though we were having a great time, we were more or less exploding with horniness.

When we got back, we got tested at the youth medical clinic and they told us we had herpes. Apparently the small blisters we had were obvious signs.

Daniel had caught genital herpes, which, obviously, is the form of herpes that affects the genitals. The most common form of herpes is herpes on or around the mouth, or what we often call cold sores. While this type of herpes (HSV-1) can spread to the genitals through oral sex, it is harder to get genital herpes (HSV-2) on the mouth through oral sex. If a person has HSV-1 on the genitals, they don't usually get it as badly or have outbreaks as often as people who have genital herpes caused by HSV-2. It is also harder to spread HSV-1 through genital contact.

Genital Warts

In ancient Rome, people thought that genital warts were spread through men having sex with boys. In fact, like most STIs, genital warts spread mostly through sexual contact, no matter who you are having sex with.

Genital warts are caused by a virus called the Human Papilloma Virus (HPV). There are many different types of HPV that affect the genital area. There are low-risk and high-risk forms of the virus. The low-risk types cause genital warts. The high-risk types cause cancer.

The problem is that men can carry the high-risk types of HPV on their penises and not know it — and there is no test for it. Generally, it's not a problem for the guy with the virus, but it can be a problem for his partner(s). Some types of HPV can affect a woman's cervix and may cause cervical cancer. Cervical cancer can be prevented through a simple test called a Pap test, which all girls should get regularly once they start having sex. People receiving anal intercourse who contract HPV may also be at risk for anal cancer.

HIV

When I was little I heard my parents talking about AIDS. It sounded horrible the way they talked about it in hushed, tight voices, and it scared me.

HIV and AIDS were discovered in 1982 by American and French scientists. Within a few short years, the fear of the virus and the virus itself had spread over the entire world. In North America, mostly gay men and intravenous drug users were affected at first. But soon, the disease spread to heterosexuals and people who didn't use drugs, including hemophiliacs and people receiving blood transfusions. Now, worldwide, the primary cause of transmission is heterosexual sex.

At the beginning, no one really knew how the virus spread,

HIV Fact Sheet

How It Works: The virus destroys your body's white blood cells and makes copies of itself in the process. Eventually, so many white blood cells are wiped out that the body's immune defenses are severely weakened. Because of this, people infected with HIV become vulnerable to any number of minor and major infectious diseases. When HIV progresses to this stage, it's called AIDS.

HIV Is Spread:
- through unprotected vaginal or anal intercourse with an infected person
- by sharing infected needles
- from a mother to her fetus in utero, or to her baby during childbirth or through breastfeeding

If a person has an untreated STI, it is easier to get infected with HIV.

Men who have unprotected oral sex with men who also have syphilis can spread – or get – HIV much more easily. So some things put you at higher risk for getting HIV:
- untreated STIs
- unprotected intercourse, especially with someone who is in the first three months of their infection
- receiving unprotected anal sex

Symptoms: Usually you don't feel any symptoms during the first few years after infection. If a person does get symptoms in the early stages, they are a lot like the flu – swollen lymph nodes, muscle aches, fatigue, fever – or sometimes skin rash and diarrhea. Once the symptoms begin, they can range from fatigue, coughing and night sweats to high fever, pneumonia, blindness, organ failure and rapid weight loss.

Testing: Blood test. For an accurate test result, it's best to wait until three months after infection. Your blood is tested for the antibodies to the virus, not the virus itself.

Treatment: As yet, there is no cure. But there are drugs called anti-retrovirals or ARVs that put the brakes on the virus and strengthen the immune system.

Related Diseases: There are a number of diseases associated with AIDS called opportunistic infections, which strike when the body's natural defenses have been broken down. These include pneumonia and some forms of cancer.

and a lot of people were afraid of catching it from kissing or public bathrooms. Now we know better. Today there are medications called anti-retrovirals (ARVs) that slow the progress of the AIDS virus once someone has become infected. However, the effectiveness of and access to those drugs is still limited, especially in developing countries.

Chapter 11
The First Time

The virgin talk usually gets started some time around the beginning of high school. Tom has apparently screwed a whole bunch of girls and people say that Petra has really gotten around. With each week that passes it seems like another person has "done it," and at some point in the midst of all the gossip and boasting, you start wondering where you stand. You don't want to be like that guy in your class who'll probably never get laid. Most likely, you want to be like the ones who are getting some, or at least getting close. But so far it hasn't even been an option. On the one hand, you want to. On the other hand, you worry about it a lot. Will I be good enough? What if I make an idiot of myself? How do I learn how to have sex when I've never had a chance to practice? Is it ever going to happen to me?

It's easy to turn virginity into way too big an issue. If you do, it can almost feel like you're not a functioning human being until you've had sex. The worst-case scenario is that you stress out and rush into things. That's never good, because certain things take time. Often, sex happens when you least expect it.

Other people are romantically inclined and want the first time to be sweet and perfect. They would rather wait for "the one" and dream up pictures of what it's going to be like. But there are no guarantees. So if you wait for everything to fall into place, to be wonderful and lovely the first time, you could easily be disappointed.

Remind yourself that your first time is not a sexuality entrance exam, and it's definitely not pass/fail. You shouldn't count on being a pro.

How was your first time?

Erika, 15
I'm a virgin. I'm a bit nervous about my sexual debut, but not too worried. Most of all, I feel a lot of anticipation. At least I'm not scared. Sometimes it bothers me that I'm a virgin, and then I just want to get it over with. But sometimes I want to be ready for it to be special.

Karen, 18
I was seventeen. It was on my aunt's couch. Actually, it was really good. The sex act itself was short, but it was amazing anyway. He was my first real love. We had known each other for a few weeks. It was a good start to my sex life.

Victor, 17
I was fifteen. It was with a friend who was a girl. We weren't in love. We just ended up doing it after having a couple of drinks. I had been attracted to her at times, but mostly she was just a buddy. Afterwards we decided that it was just something that happened once. We didn't want to ruin our friendship.

We were at her cottage with a few other friends. We got a buzz and went walking across a field with our friends. She took the initiative and kissed me. Our friends kept walking and we just stood under the trees and kissed for a while. Then we went inside and had sex.

I was very nervous about my first time, but that evaporated once it finally happened. I wanted to get rid of my virginity, even though I insisted to my friends that I was saving myself. Sex is pretty nice, but it's not as mind-blowing and important as everyone says it is.

Evelyn, 17
I was sixteen. It was confusing. Everything went wrong. Because I was in love, head over heels in love. We weren't going out. It happened very quickly, and then he left me and everything turned weird. I never knew if he was interested in me, because sometimes he would ignore me and sometimes he would pay attention to me. We only had sex once. I guess it was a traumatic experience, and it kind of disturbed the way I felt about sex. Since then, I have been able to enjoy sex, but it's been difficult. I find it hard to relax since I'm freaked out about the consequences. Will I be abandoned again?

I don't know what I was thinking, exactly, but I know that I was interested in him and that he gave me false hope after it happened. He also talked a lot about me to his friends.

I have a hard time trusting people, especially guys. Recently I've met a really wonderful person. It's a girl and I really trust her. Deep down I always thought that I was bisexual, but she's my first girlfriend. It's easier to trust girls, because they think more about emotions than guys. At least, that's my experience.

Carl, 17
I am a proud virgin and I don't find it hard to tell my friends and classmates. I want to wait for true love. All my friends in grade twelve were really surprised when I told them I was a virgin. I feel like maybe I should do something about it, but I don't really want to. I don't feel especially nervous about the first time. If you know each other and both people want to, everything should be fine.

What Does It Mean to Lose Your Virginity?
When we talk about losing our virginity we mostly mean vaginal

penetration — that is, the penis in the vagina. But isn't that a bit narrow-minded? Yes, it is. It excludes gays and lesbians. They lose their virginity, too, even if they don't penetrate or get penetrated vaginally. That's why it's not really valid to say the penis has to be in the vagina for it to be "losing your virginity." One person might think getting a hand job is enough to make him no longer a virgin, and another guy might think licking his girl is crossing into non-virgin territory. Really, it's up to each person to decide what it takes to turn the page on their virginity. Still, a lot of guys consider the first time they have sexual intercourse as losing their virginity, so we will focus on that in this chapter.

Foreplay

Suddenly it seems like it's actually going to happen. You are going to have sex. At this point it's common for guys to become impatient: it's as if you want to just stick it in as quickly as possible. In the worst case scenario, you might totally forget one of the best things of all: caressing, kissing, nibbling and cuddling. Hands on thighs, lips on earlobes – it's what we call foreplay. Foreplay is a pretty stupid and badly named concept: because our world is so fixated on penetration, it implies a prelude to intercourse. But not everything is about sticking it in. There are plenty of other amazing things to do. And during foreplay, you may not know yet if you are going to have intercourse.

It's true, however, that foreplay and the kissing, nibbling and touching that goes with it have their advantages for leading up to sex. People need different amounts of time to get turned on enough for sex. When girls are excited, they get wet – and without that, having sex with a girl is painful and pointless. That's why it's great to neck for a while first, to build up the horny feeling. Besides, sex is even better when you are at the peak of horniness and anticipation.

Nakedness

As a kid, you are completely unaware and uninhibited about being naked. You run around, penis dangling, with no shame whatsoever. You have no problem being naked in the bath around your family, and around other little kids, too, at daycare or when you go swimming at the lake. Then everything changes. All of a sudden, guys and girls have separate changing rooms, and you learn to carefully shield your genitals from others, especially those of the opposite sex. So when you're finally about to have sex, it's been so long since you hung out naked in front of someone else that taking your clothes off in front of each other can feel awkward. Doubts start setting in somewhere in the back of your mind. Is my dick too small? Am I too skinny? Am I even remotely attractive?

But at the same time, nakedness is one of the most beautiful things there is. It's all about wanting someone so much that you can let go of all your self-consciousness. Even hugging each other naked is an incredible feeling. Belly against belly, pelvis against pelvis, chest against chest.

Sure, it can feel strange and uncomfortable, but you won't need to worry much about your body or your penis. Imagine that you are really interested in a girl or a guy. Just looking at that person makes you tingle. Someone can have great style when they're dressed, but you have a desire to get closer. There's no way you're going to be disappointed when the other person's clothes come off. You're not going to think, what's wrong with that person's thighs, vagina or shoulders? Instead you'll probably feel elated and even more turned on. That's exactly the same way that the girl or guy who wants to take your clothes off is going to feel. Nobody is going to judge you or feel let down by your nakedness. Everything will be much more fun if you manage to turn down the nerves. Try to just relax and enjoy.

When Are You Mature Enough to Have Sex?

When I was in middle school, I clearly remember thinking, when are you old enough to have sex? Do you have to be eighteen, or maybe even older? I was readying myself for a long wait. I still don't know the answer, because the truth is, there is no easy answer.

The age of consent is the minimum age at which a person is considered legally capable of giving informed consent to contracts or activities regulated by law, including sexual acts. In Canada, this age of consent to sexual activity is fourteen (it is eighteen in cases involving exploitation, such as prostitution and pornography, or when the older person has authority over the younger, or the younger is in a position of dependency on the older), but even people who are under fourteen can't be punished by law for having sex if the older partner is less than two years older. In the United States, the age of consent varies widely from state to state, but across North America, it is generally very unusual for anyone to be charged for consensual sexual activity as long as they are within about two years of each other in age.

The truth is that, the law aside, sexual maturity varies from individual to individual. Of course, it's impossible to claim that everyone is ready for sex at a specific age, just like you can't say that everyone under a specific age isn't ready.

Even as a child, you are a sexual being. Yes, children can get turned on and fall in love. But that doesn't mean that little boys and girls can start a sexual relationship with someone, even with a person their own age. They are still too immature and dependent on their parents, and they haven't yet learned what having sexual relations with others entails. Children are not yet able to read other people's feelings or take care of themselves or others. As children grow, they slowly learn about human relationships, which is what it means to mature. And when a boy or a girl has come far enough in his or her development, she/he will be ready for sex. By that time, he or she will have learned, among other things, that you can't use or abuse others or allow others to use or abuse you.

You can't hurt others or force them to do things against their will. Of course we don't walk around constantly thinking about these things when we are growing up, but one day, the knowledge is with us, and we have matured.

If you were to spend time trying to figure out if you are mature enough to have sex, you probably wouldn't get very far. Being aware of your own maturity level is really tough. But you will probably feel it when you are ready for sex. The important thing is that you listen to yourself. Try to shake off the expectations or pressure of the outside world. Your own feelings are the most important part.

Stephen, 16

I think I've longed to get rid of my virginity since I was like six years old or something. But when it was finally happening, I didn't want it that much. On the other hand, it did feel so amazing and cool, even though it was pretty early for me. I had just turned fourteen, and the virgin talk had already started circulating among the guys at school. I hooked up with a girl who was a year older than I was, and who I'd never hung out with before. She was in love with me, but I didn't know it at the time.

We had gone to a park to hang out after a party, and it got to be too late for me to make it home on the bus, so I asked if I could stay at her place. It was a practical thing at the time: I wasn't even thinking about sex. So I called and told my parents I was staying at a friend's place and told them her name. On the way home, she asked if I wanted to have sex with her, and I was shocked but happy, and I said yes. She was a virgin, too. When we got home to her mom's place, her mom was still out at dinner. It was a great place, with paintings everywhere — she told me her mom was a painter.

We were both pretty buzzed, and we felt weird. After a while, we went to her room and lay down on the bed. It was, like, really awkward lying there trying to get things going. And it was very dark in there, too — she wanted it pitch black.

I was surprised at how far down on the vagina the actual opening is. It still surprises me. In the dark, the vagina becomes this sort of labyrinth. I guess she was a bit nervous because she clammed up and didn't help. So in the silence, I felt around down there in vain, thinking that this was a really bad idea and I should've just headed home. But finally, I found my way inside. Apparently the pain was brutal for her. Actually, it was not nice at all. The penetration didn't last very long; I really just wasn't that into it. And the condom was causing me some problems.

The next morning, my dad called my cell wondering where the hell I was, since I was late for hockey practice. He was really mad that I hadn't called earlier. He kept questioning me about the girl, asking if my new girlfriend was going to make me screw even more things up. "She's not my girlfriend," I thought — but I felt like I couldn't say it in front of her. Then I said goodbye to her. Talk about uncomfortable, since we barely even knew each other. Even arriving at practice late and having the coach yell at me was more appealing than staying there with her. Later on when I got home, the weird feeling caught up with me, and I felt strange and ambivalent about things. After a while it shifted into a nicer I-finally-lost-my-virginity feeling. For a long time afterwards, though, I was really worried because it felt like I hadn't enjoyed the sex. I even started to tell myself that I was gay. I walked around getting ready for life as a homosexual. That lasted quite a while, because it was a long time before I had sex again. That period was hard, because I longed to be close to girls, but I was also scared that I would end up in the same situation. But the next time I tried, it worked out.

How Do You Do It When You Do It?

One of the most common questions guys ask is: how do you find your way inside the girl? I wondered the same thing myself. That's partly why I planned to get ready for my first time by watching porn. But in reality, porn is one of the reasons that guys are so worried about not finding their way. Because in the porn world, the man is always the aggressor who takes charge and makes all the moves. He always finds the right way while the woman stays pretty passive. That's not the way it works in the real world. There are two of you having sex, so you actually don't need to worry. The girl you're with knows where her vaginal opening is. And it's much more suave to ask for help than to bring a manual with you to navigate through the big moment.

Some people get so psyched when they find the right way that they get carried away and push it in as quickly as they can. That can mean serious pain for the girl. You have to push your penis in gradually, a little bit at a time, and keep checking with the girl to make sure your penis feels okay in her vagina and that she wants to keep going.

Afterwards

Life is not like a fairy tale. You imagine feeling overwhelmingly great after sex, and wanting to lie there touching and kissing and savoring the moment. Sometimes it is like that, but not always. And there's nothing weird about that. When sexual excitement is at its most intense, you are very vulnerable. Being naked, turned on and experiencing pleasure means showing the other person the most private parts of yourself. When the orgasms are over and the intense exhilaration dies down a bit, it can feel like coming down from a big high. Regular things can suddenly feel dreary or awkward. The kisses might not taste as great any more. You might be at a loss for what to say. The doubts may reappear. Just remember that you're probably not the only one feeling that way, and do your best to relate to your partner warmly and directly.

Chapter 12
Orgasm

Omigod. It's getting closer. Getting crazy hot. The point of no return. Everything feels incredible. The intense convulsions in your groin are beyond your control. The sperm squirts out and a contented feeling spreads throughout your entire body.

Orgasm means sexual climax. For guys it's pretty easy to get there. But it can feel different from guy to guy and from orgasm to orgasm. Sometimes your whole body is in on it, and it feels like a huge tidal wave. Often it just feels like a big yawn or a nice stretch after you wake up.

People love talking about orgasms. They're discussed on the Internet, on TV, in magazines and in locker rooms. It's easy to get a little obsessed about bringing your partner to orgasm, and to become convinced that nothing else is as important. Some guys are so focused on giving their girlfriend multiple orgasms that they forget about their own pleasure while they're having sex. When the person you're having sex with doesn't come, it can feel like a failure. But you shouldn't have to feel that way. The idea that we only enjoy sex if we're having orgasms is pretty ridiculous.

A certain percentage of girls do in fact have a hard time reaching orgasm. Some girls never do, and others start to orgasm at a later stage in life. No one is born with the ability to reach orgasm. That's something you figure out through practice; for example, by masturbating. But it's also about being outspoken and open-minded about what feels good. So encourage your partner to tell you what they think will bring them to orgasm rather than trying to figure it out on your own. Since it's often easier for guys to reach orgasm, your female partner might need a bit longer or a more specific kind of touching to get there. Just ask her. And as always, there are plenty of exceptions to the rule.

Remember that it's not just your responsibility to satisfy your partner — it takes two to tango, as the saying goes. Obviously you want to bring pleasure to the person you're having sex with, but just because you don't know exactly what to do to bring them to orgasm doesn't mean you're a failed lover or anything close. The reasons for a girl not reaching orgasm vary from girl to girl, and can have to do with things you can't control. She may not have learned the best spots and what kind of touching she needs; she may feel self-conscious or pressured; or she may have a hard time getting turned on enough or feel weird about telling you what turns her on. So a sense of fun, mutual curiosity and discovery are your best tools in helping her figure out what pleasures her.

The two most common ways for girls to reach orgasm are through clitoral stimulation and through stimulation of the G-spot, which is on the front vaginal wall. So try some things out together, like rubbing her clit during intercourse, or having her on top so she can find her G-spot and rub it with your penis. But just because you touch the clitoris or the G-spot doesn't mean she will have an instant orgasm. They don't work like buttons that fire off automatically. For many girls, we're talking more like rubbing for several minutes, gentle and light to the touch.

And remember that it's not all about having an orgasm. Maybe your lover will come, maybe not. It sounds like a cliché, but the main thing is that it feels good for you and for the person you're with. Sex isn't like a race where the whole payoff is in the final lap. When it comes to sex, bliss is in every lap and around every unpredictable corner. It's not about achieving, just enjoying.

Coming Too Early

I think it's happened to every sexually active man who has walked the earth. And it's most guys' worst fear. Blowing your load too early. Premature ejaculation. In our society, guys are subject to quite a bit of pressure: you're supposed to have skill, technique and knowledge about how to satisfy your partner. So, many guys think that coming too early is a big embarrassment. They're afraid their partner is going to think they're a loser and feel cheated out of their orgasm. But it's not quite as bad as it's made out to be. Most people know it can happen and that it's not the end of the world. As I've already mentioned, sex is so much more than the penis-in-vagina routine: after all, you have hands, a tongue, lips and a whole bunch of other perfectly useful limbs. So if you and your partner want to keep going, just move right along and keep making out or try oral sex.

I do have some tricks you can use to stave off premature ejaculation, though. On the way to orgasm, once you cross a certain threshold, the orgasm is coming and there's no stopping it. When you're masturbating, practice stopping for a rest just before you reach that threshold. Then you can start again and bring yourself close to the threshold again. By figuring out where the threshold is, you can learn to develop better control over the road to your orgasm during intercourse, too. Another variation is the stop and start method. When you have sex with someone and feel the orgasm coming, stop what you're doing (kissing, oral sex, intercourse). Once you feel like everything has calmed down, start again.

Faking It

There seem to be a lot of guys who worry about this. Could she be faking? Is she just lying there pretending to come when I'm trying my best down here? I don't have any statistics or scientific studies that show how widespread fake orgasms are among human females, so I can't give you a straight answer. But I can tell you some reasons why I think some girls fake it. There are girls who don't want to hurt the guy's feelings. She thinks he will feel like a failure if she doesn't come, and so she fakes it. An even worse variation is that the two of them have never figured out what feels good for her, and she fakes orgasm so she can get the sex over with because she's not enjoying herself.

Some of you are probably wondering if you can tell a fake orgasm from a real one by listening to the girl's breathing or something. The truth is, it can be very hard to tell if someone is faking it, even if you know the person very well, because there are as many orgasm sounds as there are people. If she sounds like she's coming, she probably is. Wasting valuable pleasure-time on acting like the orgasm-police is hardly worthwhile. Think positive.

Chapter 13
Other Good Things to Know About Sex

There are some things I just don't get. For example, I don't get why there are people who try to talk other people into making out or having sex. The guys who continue touching, begging and pleading to go a bit further, even after the "no" has been communicated, clear as day. If you do manage to nag your way into having sex, it means you've "succeeded" in having sex with someone who actually doesn't want to. Meaning that it's not a very pleasant thing to "succeed" at. Not very pleasant at all.

Being able to say no is really important. I'm not much for overemphasizing rules when it comes to sex. But one thing you should definitely be proficient in before you get into sex is saying no. If you can't draw this clear and simple boundary for yourself and respect the same boundary for those you are with, you aren't ready for sexual relations. "No" is great, because it leaves no room for guessing or debating.

When it comes to sex, you can't make demands. There's nothing that says that the person who got into the game has to continue or finish playing. If someone asks you to stay over or even says they want to have sex with you, it doesn't mean you have the right to expect sex. Everyone has the right to change their mind any time they want about having or not having sex. It doesn't matter if it's a one-night stand or a more committed relationship: sex can never be taken for granted.

But just because your partner has said no once doesn't mean that you will never make out, have intercourse, or do whatever the person has said no to. And you can always ask why — but don't expect or demand an answer. Also, it might be better to avoid having the "why" conversation when you've just been turned down. If you're lying there with a hard-on asking why she/he doesn't want to do it, it can seem like pressure or like you're questioning his or her decision. That kind of reaction is very unpleasant. Wait until your hard-on is gone, and then wait a bit longer. Having a conversation about desire when you're horny doesn't work very well.

Getting a "no" isn't easy. Different people mean different things by it. If your partner is laughing, "No, no, no," and grabbing your penis at the same time, the person probably doesn't want to stop. But you need to pay attention and check to make sure that they don't mean "no." If you are lying with someone on the couch and they say no when you get close to the top of their jeans, you can draw an important conclusion without checking further: this person doesn't want me to unbutton her/his jeans or get too close to that area. It could be that she/he will want to go there five minutes later, but it's not your role to investigate it further. When someone says no, do a quick situation analysis: is she/he saying no to all of it, or just something specific? If it's the latter, just slow way down. Don't try what they said no to again. The person who has said no will need to take the initiative in that area from here on in.

At some point you might meet someone who hasn't gotten the hang of saying no yet. In these cases, you'll need to interpret other, smaller signals. The body has its own way of saying no. If someone you're with suddenly stiffens, that's an obvious sign. A person who is confident in their desire rarely goes stiff as a board. Another possible warning, if you're with a girl, might be that she's not wet. It's true that some girls get wetter than others, but if the vagina feels pretty dry, it makes sense to slow down or back up before you go any further. Keep in mind that on a physical level, lubrication is necessary to minimize painful friction in the vagina.

As I said, it's not enough to be good at understanding and accepting a "no." You have to be good at saying it yourself, too. It doesn't have to be scary, hurtful or dramatic. If it hurts when someone stimulates your nipples too hard, you have to tell them. And if you don't want to have sex, you're allowed to bow out, no matter what. In other areas, like work and studying, it can be reasonable to forget about your own immediate needs for awhile. But with sex, it's different: no one gets to make you do anything you don't want to do.

Trophy Collecting

We humans are pretty fond of collecting things. Most of us have collections like hockey cards, stamps and bottle caps crowding our drawers and basements. Then there are the people who collect things to show off how great and cool they are. Like heads of animals they have killed. That's called trophy collecting. Some people subscribe to the warped view that sex is a game of conquest, just like hunting for moose or antelope heads. They see making out and sex as failures and successes. Often, the hotter and harder to get a person is, the more their trophy is worth. But sex shouldn't be like a hunting game where you prove to yourself or others how skilled you are. You're having sex with a person, and you can't collect or own people. I don't mean that it's wrong or bad to make out or have sex with lots of people. But since sex is about an interaction between people, it's twisted to look at it as trophy collecting or another notch in your belt.

If you make it your goal to have sex with as many people as you can, be prepared to catch yourself pulling some stupid moves to get there. Think about hunting: it's not easy. You don't tell the moose, "Come here so I can kill you and hang your head on my wall." You're more likely to invest lots of time camouflaging yourself, followed by hours of trying to remain invisible. People who collect trophies in the form of sex partners are just as likely to lie, sneak around or otherwise deceive people to get their precious trophies. They say what they need to say to get laid. And dishonesty makes sex much less alluring than it can be. So what do I say to the trophy collectors? Everything is much better if you see your partner as a person. Honesty is the only way to really be able to enjoy the mutual pleasure sex has to offer.

SBF

Sex and making out don't have to have anything to do with love. There are some obvious advantages to having sex with someone you're in love with and/or in a relationship with. But there are also pros to petting and sex without love. Sex and making out don't need to be beautiful, passionate or sweet. They come in all kinds of variations. In the middle of a make-out session, you're not necessarily thinking about how much you love the person. Sometimes it's hard to tell — is it your heart or your groin that's throbbing?

SBF is short for sex between friends. It can mean two things. On the one hand, it can refer to an understanding with a friend that you'll meet up once in awhile just to make out or have sex. You know right away there's the likelihood of sex whenever the person's phone number comes up on your cell display. Or it can mean you have a friend with whom you sometimes have sex or make out. In both cases, the fact that you're not in love is the whole point. Some people are well-suited to SBF-type relations. For others, the absence of butterflies and tingling leaves them unsatisfied. There are SBF arrangements that work, although most of them don't last long. In many cases, one of the parties falls in love. And if the love is unrequited — as it often is — it means a quick and painful, or in some cases, slow and devastating, end to the friendship.

When Friendship Turns into Sex

A typical scenario is that you are close friends with someone, you hang out and do fun things together, you support each other when you're going through rough times, and you cheer each other up when you feel low. Maybe you've comforted each other with hugs and crashed at each others' places.

Then one night you're watching a movie or hanging out after a party, just chatting, and after the usual hug, your lips happen to meet. So you go for it: kiss, make out, maybe even have sex. Most likely, this "mistake" will change your relationship with this person in some way. If it becomes too weird or embarrassing to see the person, it might even mean the end of the friendship. How do you look at each other without being constantly reminded of what happened? How do you hang out on the couch or hug each other goodbye without it bringing up the sexual feelings you may or may not have for this person? Or it could be that you both enjoyed it so much, you keep going — either through occasional make-out sessions or by starting an actual relationship. The least common possibility is that both people shrug their shoulders and move right along as if nothing happened.

Sex and making out usually fall outside the boundaries of friendship because, in reality, it's hard to combine friendship and a sexual relationship. Often it's confusing because it involves different sets of feelings. You might start to feel jealousy if your friend sits close to some other hottie at a party or at school. Feelings like that should be a clear indication to you that things have gone too far.

As always, there are shining exceptions. There are friendships that can withstand "slip-ups," and friends who feel good about having sex with each other — or at least not bad about it.

The best approach, as always, is to talk to your friend. Together you can go through what really happened between the two of you, and decide what type of relationship you both want for the future.

Oral Sex

Oral means "with the mouth," and sex means "having to do with sexual activity." It's not rocket science: oral sex means having sex with your mouth. Some people think oral sex is more intimate than other kinds of sex, like intercourse, whereas others feel the opposite is true.

There was a wide variety of reactions among the public to the most famous oral sex of our time: the affair involving Monica Lewinsky and Bill Clinton. When their relationship was discovered, some people defended Clinton, claiming that oral sex wasn't "real" sex and therefore Clinton hadn't in fact been unfaithful. After the Lewinsky affair, the Oval Office in the White House has often been jokingly referred to as the Oral Office.

How Do You Give Oral Sex?

We've already covered how you give guys oral sex in the chapter on homosexuality, but we still have to cover how you give a girl oral sex. In other words, how you lick her.

Licking someone is a great way to get to know how her vagina works. You can't get much closer than that. Of course intercourse brings you close, too, but your penis can't taste or smell anything.

That's probably one of the main reasons that girls sometimes feel self-conscious about being licked: they worry about smelling bad to their partner. Having a shower together beforehand can make them more comfortable. But also, let them know that you are into exploring their smell and taste — from my experience, and from most guys' point of view, vaginas look, taste and smell fine.

The first vagina-licking ground rule is: start carefully — very few girls enjoy having a guy throw himself at their vagina with a tongue that is as hard as rock and as fast as a propeller. After that, it's all about feeling your way, since each girl is a different story. Start with soft tongue fluttering around the clitoral hood, then gently separate the outer labia with your tongue or fingers, and explore the inside. Suck loosely and try making small, fast, soft circles. If you need inspiration, there's a classic technique called "tongue-ABC" that involves making letters with your tongue around the clitoris.

The second ground rule is to listen and pay attention to your partner's response — her reaction should tell you whether you are going in the right direction. If not, the best route is to simply ask her: if you give her the chance, she will describe the tongue action that works for her. It's better not to move around too quickly; keep at it for several minutes in one area if it seems to be working. The practice-makes-perfect rule applies with oral sex, too! And feel free to express your own pleasure: the girl will relax knowing that you are enjoying yourself. Last thing to remember: while some girls take longer than others, oral sex is not a marathon. It's not the man who keeps going the fastest and longest who wins. If you've been going for longer than fifteen minutes, chances are you could be licking in a better spot or with a different rhythm.

Anal Sex

Until quite recently, anal sex was considered "unnatural." Since it didn't have anything to do with procreation, it was seen as sinful. Today, there is a revival of some of the fear surrounding anal sex, but in a different context. People are talking about the trend that some women and girls feel pressured to have anal sex because their partner is influenced by porn. I don't want to take a stand for or against anal sex here, but I do think you should know what it's about in reality — as opposed to in the world of porn — before you and your partner get into it.

Anal sex involves stimulation in and around the anus. There are lots of variations of anal sex. You can finger, lick, penetrate and much more. Licking the anus is also called rimming. Anal sex feels good because there are many sensitive nerve endings in and around the anus. It can also be exciting because it feels forbidden and a little kinky. And specifically for men, it can involve stimulating the sensitive prostate gland.

When people say anal sex, they often mean anal intercourse that is, penetrating anal sex. Anal intercourse is delicate and complex. It requires a lot of mutual trust and preparation — mental and physical. And you have to be absolutely vigilant about using condoms and lots of water-based lubricant. Most important of all, you and your partner both must have the honest and open desire to try it out. Usually, it's best to have quite a bit of sexual experience under your belt before you and your partner have anal intercourse.

Before engaging in anal intercourse with others, it makes sense to test it out on yourself to find out what it feels like. Even if you're straight, it doesn't mean you're definitely doing the penetrating just because you're a guy. Your girlfriend can insert a finger, a dildo or another object into your anus just as easily as you can penetrate her with your penis or something else. Use water-based lube to insert a finger or another object into yourself while you masturbate. Try to relax and go in a tiny bit at a time. In men, about ten centimeters (four inches) into the anus, the prostate gland bulges into the rectum. It's about the size of a walnut. Many guys find pressure against the prostate gland feels great, and some guys orgasm just from stimulating the prostate. The gland is located on the front side of the rectum, that is, on the same side as the stomach.

Fingers are usually great tools to use during anal sex of any kind, so an important ground rule is trimming your nails so they are short. Long nails can hurt, and they can damage the sensitive rectal mucous membrane.

Anal intercourse is far from being something that everyone enjoys. It can be very painful if you don't go about it right. Since the anus doesn't have any natural lubrication, you have to use plenty of water-based lube. Make sure you buy a good brand of water-based lube from the drugstore. A good way to prepare for anal intercourse is to put lube on the fingers and stroke your partner's anus. Then slide a finger into the anus using lots of lube. Go in a little bit at a time. When the person being penetrated feels ready and is as relaxed as possible, very slowly insert a dildo or the penis. Some girls find they can relax and enjoy it more if they masturbate at the same time.

When you have any kind of sex, it's important to listen for cues from your partner. Having sex with another person requires that you pick up on your partner's signals continuously so that you can stop when it no longer feels good for her or him. When it comes to anal intercourse, it's extra important or things can go wrong very easily. The best approach is to let the person being penetrated take control, directing when and how much anal penetration they can handle.

It's also crucial to think about how you both can stay protected. Using a condom is the best way to effectively protect both of you from STIs that easily spread in the rectum. The last ground rule you have to stick to is to carefully clean any objects or body parts with soap and water right after engaging in anal sex or anal intercourse — that includes your hands, mouth or penis. Doing this is especially important before you move on to other kinds of sex. You also have to change your condom as soon as it has been used in anal sex.

Aftermath

This is the end of the book, but hopefully the beginning of a great friendship. Maybe you are already good buddies with sex and love — if not, it will probably happen soon. Having a sex life and a love life is about incredible feelings and experiences, but it's also about sadness and frustration.

You will live it all.

Before you slam this book shut and head out into the world, I want to remind you about something. You don't need to worry too much about making a fool of yourself in sex and love. My high school biology teacher once said, "The first sexual experience is like driving a car for the first time: it's nerve-wracking and technically, far from perfect; sometimes you even end up in the ditch. But it's fantastic fun to try, and you learn quickly."

The best method when it comes to sex is trial and error. Do what you feel like doing. And as the Bible says, "Do unto others as you would have them do unto you." That's a great guideline for sex as well as the rest of your life.

It's been great having you along for the ride.

Come back again — and good luck with everything.

For Further Information

Books

Bass, Ellen and Kate Kauffman. *Free Your Mind: The Book for Gay, Lesbian and Bisexual Youth and Their Allies*. New York: Harper Collins, 1996.

Beauvoir, Simone de. *The Second Sex*. New York, Toronto: Alfred A. Knopf, 1993.

Bell, Ruth. *Changing Bodies, Changing Lives*. 3rd ed. New York: Three Rivers Press, 1998.

Kinsey, Alfred C., Wardell B. Pomeroy and Clyde E. Martin. *Sexual Behavior in the Human Male*. Philadelphia: W. B. Saunders Co., 1948.

Nathan, Debbie. *Pornography*. Groundwork Guides. Toronto: Groundwood Books / House of Anansi Press, 2007.

Pavanel, Jane. *The Sex Book*. Montreal: Lobster Press, 2001.

Savin-Williams, Ritch C. *The New Gay Teenager*. Cambridge, MA: Harvard University Press, 2005.

Internet

Advocates for Youth of Toronto
  www.youthresource.com
Answer, Rutgers University
  www.sexetc.org
The Coalition for Postive Sexuality (CPS)
  www.positive.org
Go Ask Alice! / Health Services at Columbia
  www.goaskalice.columbia.edu
Parents, Families and Friends of Lesbians and Gays
  www.pflag.org
Planned Parenthood Federation of America
  www.teenwire.com
Planned Parenthood of Toronto
  www.ppt.on.ca
The Sexual Health Network
  www.sexualhealth.com

Videos

Baines, Paul. *Shoulder to Shoulder: Men and Vulnerability*. DVD. Toronto: MediaMindful, 2006. www.mediamindful.ca.

Katz, Jackson. *Tough Guise: Media and the Crisis in Masculinity*. DVD/VHS. Northampton, MA: Media Education Foundation, 1999.

Acknowledgments

All of the interviews in *Sex for Guys* are authentic, but some of the names have been changed. I want to thank all those who agreed to be interviewed. And a big thank-you to my readers – you know who you are. Thanks also to Professor Claes Sundelin and Sandra Dahlén.

– Manne Forssberg

Groundwood Books would like to thank for their valuable assistance Allie Lehmann, Jude Johnston, Lyba Spring and Herbert Co from Toronto Public Health, and Gillian Watts.

Index